Arthritis & Osteoporosis

Home Exercise Guide & Workbook

Plus

Exercise Benefits & Precautions

Lost Temple Fitness & Rehab

Karen Cutler: LPTA, ACE Certified Personal Trainer,
Medical, Cancer, Arthritis &Therapeutic Exercise Specialist

Websites

LostTempleFitness.com

LostTempleNutrition.com

LostTemplePets.com

LostTempleArt.com

LostTempleFitnessCancer.com

Introduction

It has been proven that exercise and nutrition are two of the main factors that you can control for a healthy lifestyle. Many people do not know how to start or progress an exercise program. There are hundreds of pictures for beginner, intermediate and advanced exercise programs, as well as a list of equipment that you can use in the home. This also includes worksheets to help you track your exercises and progress.

The Arthritis & Osteoporosis section includes information osteoarthritis, rheumatoid arthritis and also osteoporosis, which is when the bones become brittle and fragile. This includes definitions, symptoms, precautions and exercise benefits.

This book is for:

- Those with a diagnosis of Osteoporosis, Osteoarthritis or Rheumatoid arthritis
- The beginner who has never exercised before
- The individual that has mastered the basics but wants to know how to advance to the next level.
- Pre/post rehab individuals who would like to advance or want a list of exercise programs to follow.
- The personal trainer, physical therapist, or other coaches who would like their client to have a list of exercises that can be progressed.

This book is not for or may need modification:

- Chronic or acute disorders/injury's that is not being followed by a health care professional. This book can be used in conjunction with a rehab program.
- If you are over 40 and have never exercised before, it is advised that a physician clears you first.
- Undiagnosed pain
- The person that does not feel they can safely modify their individual program, although can be used in conjunction with rehab or coaches/personal trainers.
- People with the following issues that have been cleared by an MD for an exercise program or in conjunction with rehab. These issues will be addressed in future volumes: Cardiac & Pulmonary disease, Cancer or Diabetes.

What is covered in this book?
- Arthritis Type, Affected Joints, Definition, Disease Characteristics, Increased Risks, Prevention, Exercise Tips, Modify Discontinue Exercise and Nutrition for Arthritis with Food Charts.
- Home Exercise Programs – pictures and explanations
    - Myofascial release
    - Flexibility – Stretching
    - Core Stability
    - Balance with progression to Standing Strengthening exercises
    - Strengthening
    - Lower extremity - Lying and Seated
    - Upper extremity
- Benefits and Factors to consider before starting an exercise program
- Vital signs and how to monitor exercise intensity
- Temperature – Heat and Cold
- Dehydration
- Anatomy – Anatomical Positions and Directions
- Muscles/Joint actions, Skeleton/Range of Motion
- Equipment needed for home exercise
- Warm up/cool down
- Duration, Frequency, Intensity and Primary Movement Patterns

Lost Temple Fitness

INTRODUCTION

Arthritis & Osteoporosis

See Section for Specific TOC

REFERENCES

HOME EXERCISE PROGRAM
See Section for Specific TOC

Arthritis & Osteoporosis
Benefits and Precautions for Exercising with Arthritis / Osteoporosis

Starting an exercise program with arthritis or pre-arthritis can be different than for an otherwise healthy adult. This supplement to the *Home Exercise Guide* will explain the benefits of starting an exercise program, but also some precautions or things you should not do. This will also cover some diets and foods to eat or not eat to help decrease inflammation.

- **Osteopenia** - Reduced bone mass of lesser severity than osteoporosis.

- **Osteoporosis** - A medical condition in which the bones become brittle and fragile from loss of tissue, typically as a result of hormonal changes, or deficiency of calcium or vitamin D.

- **Osteoarthritis** - Degeneration of joint cartilage and the underlying bone, most common from middle age onward. It causes pain and stiffness, especially in the hip, knee, and thumb joints.

- **Rheumatoid arthritis** - A chronic progressive disease that causes inflammation in the joints, resulting in painful deformity and immobility, especially in the fingers, wrists, feet, and ankles.

Exercise information is from: ACE – *Fitness Professionals Guide to Training Clients with Osteoarthritis / Mayo Clinic / WebMD / National Institute of Arthritis and Musculoskeletal and Skin Diseases (NISM) / National Osteoporosis Foundation (AF) / American College of Sports Medicine (ACSM) / Association of Rheumatology Health Professionals (ARHP) / MedicineNet.com*

Nutrition information is from: *Arthritis Foundation / Chewfo / US News / Mayo Clinic / David Perlmutter / Celiac Disease Foundation / Dr. Weil*

Arthritis & Osteoporosis Table of Contents

Quick Summary this Section

Types, Commonly Affected Joints & Definitions

Osteoporosis	Osteoarthritis (OA)	Rheumatoid Arthritis (RA)
TYPES		
Bone Density	Local, Degenerative	Inflammatory, Systemic, Autoimmune
COMMONLY AFFECTED JOINTS		
Hip Ribs Spine Wrist	Hands Hips Knees Spine	Cervical spine Feet Hands Knees Wrists
DEFINITION		

Osteopenia

- Osteopenia is a condition of bone that is slightly less dense than normal bone, but not to the degree of bone in osteoporosis.
- Your bones are usually at their densest when you're about 30. Osteopenia, if it happens at all, usually occurs after age 50.
- The exact age depends how strong your bones are when you're young. If they're hardy, you may never get osteopenia.
- If your bones aren't naturally dense, you may get it earlier.

Osteoporosis

- Osteoporosis is a condition characterized by a decrease in the density of bone, decreasing its strength and resulting in fragile bones.
- Osteoporosis literally leads to abnormally porous bone that is compressible, like a sponge. This disorder of the skeleton weakens the bone and results in frequent fractures (breaks) in the bones.
- Bones that are affected by osteoporosis can break (fracture) with relatively minor injury that normally would not cause a bone to fracture.
- The fracture can be either in the form of cracking (as in a hip fracture) or collapsing (as in a compression fracture of the vertebrae of the spine).
- The spine, hips, ribs, and wrists are common areas of bone fractures from osteoporosis although osteoporosis- related fractures can occur in almost any skeletal bone.

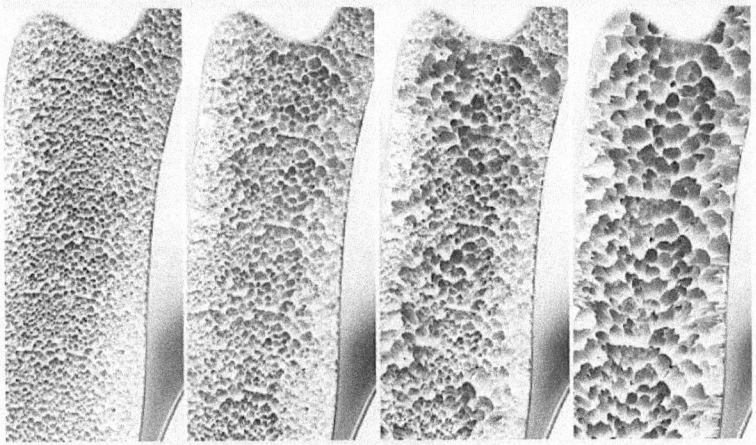

Osteoarthritis (OA)	• Osteoarthritis likely begins with the breakdown of articular cartilage, a tough material that cushions and protects the bone ends. • Cartilage allows bones to smoothly glide over one another and effectively absorb the shock of physical movement. • With OA, cartilage becomes damaged and ineffective, leaving the bones to rub against one another during movement. This process may be stimulated by high circulating levels of pro- inflammatory cytokines and other inflammatory cells. • Friction in the joint causes pain, swelling, and decreased range of motion. • Sometimes small deposits of bone, known as osteophytes, start to grow at the edge of the joint. If these osteophytes break off and float into the joint space, they can cause more pain and damage.
Rheumatoid Arthritis (RA)	• Rheumatoid arthritis is an inflammatory disease that causes pain, swelling, stiffness, and loss of function in the joints. • The body's immune system essentially turns against itself. • RA typically occurs in a symmetrical pattern. For example, when one knee or hand is involved, the other one is also involved. • The disease often affects the wrist and finger joints closest to the hand. Other body parts and systems can also be affected. (*National Institute of Arthritis and Musculoskeletal and Skin Diseases (NISM)*) • Inflammation in the synovium causes changes in the joint as well as ligament laxity and loss of strength.

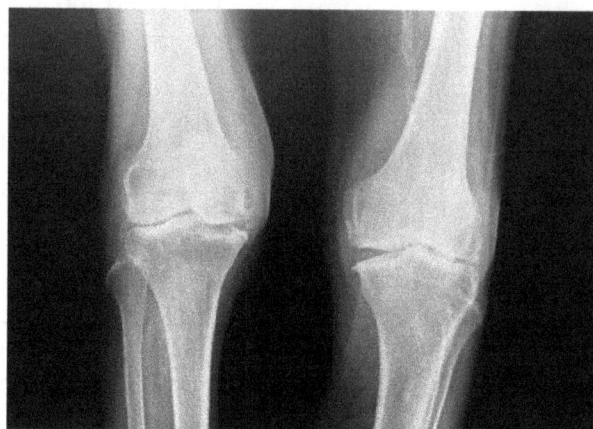

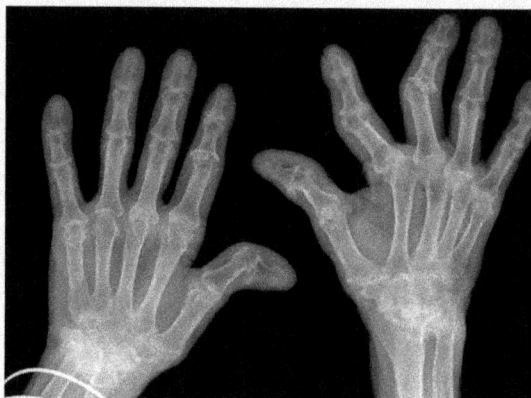

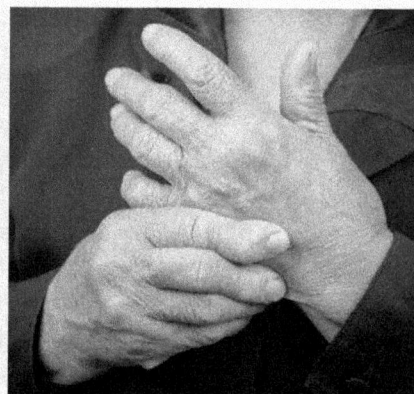

Disease Characteristics

Osteoporosis	Osteoarthritis (OA)	Rheumatoid Arthritis (RA)
There typically are no symptoms in the early stages of bone loss, but once your bones have been weakened by osteoporosis, you may have signs and symptoms that include: • Back pain, caused by a fractured or collapsed vertebra • Loss of height over time • A stooped posture • A bone fracture that occurs much more easily than expected *(Mayo Clinic)*	• Onset older age • Joint pain, swelling and stiffness after periods of inactivity or excessive use • Morning stiffness lasts less than 30 minutes • Cartilage degeneration • Grating or 'catching' sensation during joint movement • Joint instability and buckling (knee) • Bony growths at the margins of affected joint (osteophytes / bone spurs) • Loss of mechanical integrity of the joint • No visible joint changes can be seen in the spine, knee, or hip • Spurring and enlargement of finger joints (proximal and distal interphalangeal joints or PIP and DIP) can become visible • In OA of the foot, the metatarsal phalangeal (MTP) joints drop down, and the fat pad slips, causing hammer toes. This may affect shoe selection and ability to do weight-bearing exercise. 	• Onset younger age • Gradual or rapid onset of symptoms/pain • Morning stiffness over 30 minutes to several hours • Worse pain in the morning and at end of day • Primarily affects synovium and may include internal organs • Typically, small joints of hands and wrist symmetrically with ulnar deviation • "Crippling" arthritis • Red, swollen, warm, tender joints • Fatigue, fever, loss of energy, malaise • May have rheumatoid nodules • Acute & chronic inflammation and pain • Loss of joint integrity

Risks		
Osteoporosis	**Osteoarthritis (OA)**	**Rheumatoid Arthritis (RA)**

• Women more than men
• Age. Increases as we age.
• Race: White or of Asian descent
• Family History.
• Small body frames have higher risks
 	
Hormones
• Sex hormones. Reduced estrogen in menopausal women.
• Men with a gradual reduction in testosterone levels.
• Thyroid problems –increased.
• Overactive parathyroid and adrenal glands.
 	
Dietary factors
• Low calcium intake
• Decreased weight or food intake.
• Gastrointestinal surgery.
 	
Steroids and other medications used to combat or prevent:
• Seizures
• Gastric reflux
• Cancer
• Transplant rejection
 	
Medical conditions
• Celiac disease
• Inflammatory bowel disease
• Kidney or liver disease
• Cancer
• Lupus
• Multiple myeloma
• Rheumatoid arthritis
 	
Lifestyle choices
• Sedentary lifestyle.
• Excessive alcohol consumption
• Tobacco use.
	• Increasing age
	• Family History
	• Injury or overuse
	• Old joint, injuries/surgeries
	• Aging athletes
	• Muscle weakness
	• Impaired proprioception can lead to the loss of protective muscular reflexes.
	   o Reflex inhibition is a response to pain and joint effusion (swelling).
	• High bone mass
	• Disuse:
	   o Moderate physical activity decreases OA risk.
	• Overweight/Obesity – increases the mechanical load on weight bearing joints.
		• Family History
		
		• Smoking. Some studies show it also can make it progress faster and lead to more joint damage.
		
		• Obesity. You also may be able to lower your chances by losing weight, especially if you're 55 or younger.
		
		• Research shows there may be a link between RA and periodontal (gum) disease. Brush / floss and see your dentist for regular checkups.
		
		(Web MD)

Prevention

Osteoporosis	Osteoarthritis (OA)	Rheumatoid Arthritis (RA)

• **Protein**: Building blocks of bone.
 	
• **Body weight**: Being underweight increases the chance of bone loss and fractures.
  o Excess weight is known to increase the risk of fractures in your arm and wrist.
  o Maintaining an appropriate body weight is good for bones.
 	
• **Calcium.** Men and women between the ages of 18 and 50 need 1,000 milligrams of calcium a day. This daily amount increases to 1,200 milligrams when women turn 50 and men turn 70.
 	
• **Vitamin D** improves your body's ability to absorb calcium and improves bone health in other ways. People may get adequate amounts of vitamin D from sunlight. Scientists don't yet know the optimal daily dose of vitamin D for each person. A good starting point for adults is 600 to 800 international units (IU) a day, through food or supplements.
 	
• **Exercise.** Combine strength training, weight-bearing, and balance exercises.
  o Strength training helps strengthen muscles and bones in your arms and upper spine.
  o Weight-bearing exercises such as walking, jogging, running, stair climbing, skipping rope, skiing, and impact- producing sports affect mainly the bones in your legs, hips, and lower spine.
  o Balance exercises such as tai chi can reduce your risk of falling.
 	
(Mayo clinic)
	• *See Osteoporosis*
	
	• Moderate physical activity actually decreases OA risk.
	
	Weight loss.
	• For every one pound of weight loss, there is a 4 lb. reduction in the load exerted on the knee for each step taken during daily activities.
	
	• Losing as few as 11 pounds can cut the risk of developing knee OA by 50% for some women.
	
	• Weight loss of only 15 lbs. can cut knee pain in half for overweight individuals with arthritis.
		• There's no known way to prevent RA, but scientists are studying DNA markers that show that someone will develop it.
		
		• New research has shown that there is a narrow window of opportunity for early treatment that can literally stop the disease in its tracks.
		
		• Timely diagnosis and treatment can prevent the progression of RA and the associated joint destruction. *(Fitness professional guide)*
		
		*** "Ideally, you should begin treatment within 3 to 6 months of your first symptoms".
		
		(Web MD)

Exercise Tips	
Osteoporosis	**Osteoarthritis (OA)** **&** **Rheumatoid Arthritis (RA)**

High-impact weight-bearing exercises may not be safe for you if you have a higher chance of breaking a bone.
• *Talk to your doctor about your workout routine.*
• They may recommend that you focus on *low- impact* exercises that are less likely to cause fractures and still build up your bone density.
 	
These include:
• Elliptical training machines
• Low-impact aerobics
• Stair-step machines
• Walking (either outside or on a treadmill machine)
 	
Making exercise for osteoporosis safe to ensure your safety during exercise for osteoporosis, keep these guidelines in mind:
• If you already have osteoporosis, be careful of exercises that involve bending and twisting at the waist. This motion can put you at risk of fracture.
• Exercises that involve waist twisting include sit-ups and toe touches.
   o Golf, tennis, bowling, and some yoga poses also include some twisting at the waist.
• Talk to your doctor before choosing any of these activities.
	• Acute (symptoms less than 7 days)
	  o Focus on maintaining flexibility only.
	  o Do exercise daily during this phase to prevent loss of motion and contractures (muscle / tendon tightening that prevents normal movement).
	
	• Sub-acute (symptoms lasting 1-6 weeks)
	  o Work on maintaining/increasing flexibility and strength.
	  o Some cardiovascular activity can be done.
	
	• Chronic (symptoms lasting longer than 6 weeks)
	  o Focus on progressive strengthening and increase cardiovascular fitness.
	
	• Exercise daily when pain and stiffness are the least (when medications have the greatest effect and/or energy is highest).
	
	• Perform gentle ROM exercises for the affected joint(s) in both the morning (before rising) and evening to reduce stiffness.
	
	• Include all planes of movement around the affected joint and adjacent joints.
	
	• Avoid overexertion and extreme ranges of joint flexion or extension.
	
	• Modify as needed – for example, replace the Long Arc Quad (LAQ) with the Partial Arc Quad (PAQ) to decrease ROM.

Modify or Discontinue Exercise

Osteoporosis	Osteoarthritis (OA) & Rheumatoid Arthritis (RA)
• If you have osteoporosis, don't do the following types of exercises: • High-impact exercises. Activities such as jumping, running or jogging • Avoid jerky, rapid movements in general. Choose exercises with slow, controlled movements. • Bending and twisting. Exercises in which you bend forward at the waist and twist your waist, such as touching your toes or doing sit-ups, can increase your risk of compression fractures in your spine if you have osteoporosis. • Other activities that may require you to bend or twist forcefully at the waist are golf, tennis, bowling, and some yoga poses. *(Mayo clinic)*	• Joint pain/discomfort during the exercise or continuing pain (pain that lasts more than 2 hours after exercising and/or exceeds pain severity before exercise) • Respect pain—use it as a 'warning' sign. "No pain, no gain" is not true with arthritis. • Increased joint swelling/tightness immediately after or the day following activity • Decreased range of motion • Increased weakness • Altered gait following participation in a weight-bearing activity • Unusual or persistent fatigue

Osteoporosis

Exercise Types

(See Home Exercise Guide for specific terms and explanations)
Mayo Clinic / WebMD / MedicineNet.com / National Osteoporosis Foundation

Flexibility Non-Impact and Balance

- Fall prevention is especially important for people with osteoporosis.
  - Stability and balance exercises help your muscles work together in a way that keeps you more stable and less likely to fall.
  - Simple exercises such as standing on one leg or movement-based exercises such as tai chi can improve your stability and balance.
- These moves don't directly strengthen your bones. They can, though, improve your coordination, flexibility, and muscle strength. That will lower the chance that you'll fall and break a bone. You can do these every day.
- Balance exercises such as Tai Chi can strengthen your leg muscles and help you stay steadier on your feet.
  - Posture exercises can help you work against the "sloping" shoulders that can happen with osteoporosis and lower your chances of spine fractures.
- Routines such as yoga and Pilates can improve strength, balance, and flexibility.

**Some of the moves you do in these programs, including forward-bending exercises, can make you more likely to get a fracture.

Weight Bearing / Aerobic

- Weight-bearing aerobic activities involve doing aerobic exercise on your feet, with your bones supporting your weight. These types of exercise work directly on the bones in your legs, hips and lower spine to slow mineral loss. They also provide cardiovascular benefits, which boost heart and circulatory system health.
- It's important that aerobic activities, as beneficial as they are for your overall health, are not the whole of your exercise program.
- Swimming and cycling have many benefits, but they don't provide the weight-bearing load your bones need to slow mineral loss. However, if you enjoy these activities, do them.

There are two types of weight-bearing exercise: high-impact and low-impact.
High impact includes workouts like:
- Brisk walking
- Climbing stairs
- Dancing
- Hiking
- Jogging
- Jumping rope
- Step aerobics
- Tennis or other racquet sports
- Yard work, like pushing a lawnmower or heavy gardening

But be careful. High-impact weight-bearing exercises may not be safe for you if you have a higher chance of breaking a bone. Talk to your doctor about your workout routine. They may recommend that you focus on low-impact exercises that are less likely to cause fractures and still build up your bone density. These include:
- Elliptical training machines
- Low-impact aerobics
- Stair-step machines
- Walking (either outside or on a treadmill machine)

**If you're new to exercise or haven't worked out for a while, you should aim to gradually increase the amount you do until you get to 30 minutes of weight-bearing exercise per day on most days of the week.

Flexibility

- Moving your joints through their full range of motion helps you keep your muscles working well.
- Stretches are best performed after your muscles are warmed up at the end of your exercise session, for example, or after a 10-minute warm-up.
  - They should be done gently and slowly, without bouncing.
- Avoid stretches that flex your spine or cause you to bend at the waist. Ask your doctor which stretching exercises are best for you.

Examples of flexibility exercise for osteoporosis include:
- Stretches
- Tai chi
- Yoga

Resistance Exercises

Resistance means you're working against the weight of another object. Resistance helps with osteoporosis because it strengthens muscle and builds bone.

Studies have shown that resistance exercise increases bone density and reduces the risk of fractures.

Resistance exercise for osteoporosis includes:
- Free weights or weight machines at home or in the gym
- Resistance tubing that comes in a variety of strengths
- Water exercises

Osteoarthritis (OA) & Rheumatoid Arthritis (RA)
Exercise Types
See Home Exercise Guide for specific terms and explanations

Information by Arthritis Foundation (AF) / American College of Sports Medicine (ACSM) / Association of Rheumatology Health Professionals (ARHP)

Flexibility & Balance

Flexibility:
- Joint motion may be maintained by performing active range of motion exercises through the entire range, 3-5 times daily.
- Move slowly and gently through full ROM, but *not* past the point of usual pain/discomfort.
- Reduce the number of repetitions with active inflammation and avoid overstretching.
  - Move the affected joint GENTLY.
  - Use a slow, steady rhythm and *do not* bounce.
- Adapt by using self-assisted techniques (wand or pulley) to perform gentle ROM or stretching.
- A warm environment promotes elasticity.

Balance:
- The pain, stiffness, joint instability, and muscular weakness associated with OA can alter proprioception and prevent efficient, controlled and integrated movement.
- Stiff and painful movements require more energy and increase fatigue. Include static and dynamic balance by introducing progressive balance challenges:
  - Progression from double limb to single limb stance activities tiptoe walking, retro walking, and lateral walking.
- Use equipment with unsteady surfaces: rocker boards, balance discs, BOSU balls, foam cushions and rolls.
  - Start with holding the back of a chair or stable object at first when introducing and unstable surface.

Strengthening / Resistance

- Start with isometric or low-load exercises. Gradually transition to isotonic/dynamic exercises, range of motion without resistance and functional movements.
- Resistance level should first be determined by the response of the joint and *not* muscle fatigue.
- Although it is ideal to perform an exercise through the complete range of motion, it may be necessary to perform a certain strength exercise in a more limited range of motion and decrease resistance to avoid joint pain.
- If you can handle more challenging exercises in joints *not* affected by OA, adapt the program accordingly.

Progression guidelines:
- Ensure that you can easily perform an exercise correctly during at least 2 consecutive workouts.
- Increase resistance by no more than 10% each week.
- Don't change too many things at a time; if you experience joint symptoms, you'll know what may have caused the problem.
- Review posture, alignment, and body mechanics. The joint being exercised should be in line with the equipment fulcrum or biomechanical stresses may increase on an unstable/misaligned joint.
- Watch your neck/spine position, particularly during abdominal work. Keep in neutral.

Don't forget about the hands/grasp and thumb/fingers involvement.

Isometric and Isotonic

Isometric:

Isometric strengthening is appropriate for those deconditioned or with joint pain during isotonic or dynamic movement. Isometric exercise allows you to strengthen the muscle without moving the joint, minimize atrophy, maintain/increase static strength/ endurance, and improve tone to prepare for dynamic and weight-bearing activity.

- Perform each exercise at multiple angles throughout the range to simulate function.
- Intensity: Good quality contraction of the muscle (moderate to hard intensity)
- Frequency: Start with 5-10 reps daily. Proceed to 3 x 15 reps.
- Duration: Hold isometric contractions 5-10 seconds.

Isotonic (*Strengthening / Resistance above*):

Dynamic or isotonic exercises maintain/increase muscle power and endurance, simulate functional movements, enhance synovial blood flow and promote strength of bone and cartilage.

- Intensity: Start w/ light resistance (10% 1 RM) and progress to light to moderate resistance (40-60% 1 RM)
- 1 x 10; 2 x 10; 3 x 10; 3 x 15 •Frequency: 2 - 3 times per week on alternate days
- Duration: 15–30 min. Progress by first increasing repetitions (10-15 reps/exercise), then increase weight by 10% week or to pain tolerance.
- Use lower resistance bands/weights to decrease stress on joint and adjust equipment for good biomechanics
- Put weights more proximal (closer) to the joint to decrease lever arm.
- **Typical quad exercises such as full ROM knee extensions may exacerbate symptoms and contribute to further degeneration of the joint.
- Modify as needed – for example, replace the Long Arc Quad (LAQ) with the Partial Arc Quad (PAQ) to decrease ROM.

** If you have arthritis in your hands, please be careful with hand weights – may want to substitute for bands/cables.

Aerobics

Aerobic exercise is an integral part of an exercise program for individuals with osteoarthritis and is associated with the following benefits:
- Improved cardiovascular function
- Increased muscular strength and flexibility
- Improved physical and social activity levels
- Reduced fatigue
- Decreased depression and anxiety
- Decreased pain
- Decreased or unchanged disease activity

Modes of aerobic exercise that work particularly well for individuals with OA include:
- Walking
- Bicycling
- Swimming or water exercise
- Low impact aerobics/chair exercise

Intensity
- For individuals who have not exercised in over 3 months/deconditioned, start at 40-60% Heart Rate Reserve (HRR/Karvonen – see *How to Monitor HR*)
- For patients at average levels of fitness >60% HRR is appropriate. More fit individuals can tolerate higher intensity levels depending upon joint mode and the presence of joint symptoms.

Duration
- The initial phase should consist of short bouts (5-10 minutes).
- Progress to 20-30 minutes above daily activity (150 min./week of moderate intensity) to increase fitness level.
- individuals may tolerate more daily exercise by breaking it up into multiple bouts. For example, a 30-minute walk may produce knee discomfort or swelling. Two 15-minute walks may be tolerated without symptoms.
- Focus on duration before intensity.

Frequency
- 3–5 days/week–individualize based on fitness and joint response (provided the person is not in the acute phase).

Finding the Best Joint Pain Relief for You
Arthritis Foundation

Oral, Injected and Topical Medications

Disease-modifying medications. If you have an inflammatory form of arthritis such as rheumatoid arthritis (RA) or psoriatic arthritis, an important route to relieving pain is controlling the underlying disease. Fortunately, a variety of medications — many developed in recent decades or years — make disease control possible. Drugs that can control the disease process include:

- **Traditional disease-modifying antirheumatic drugs or DMARDs**, such as methotrexate or leflunomide (*Arava*).
- **Biological agents or biologics**, which are drugs genetically engineered to inhibit or modify components of the immune system, including B cells, tumor necrosis factor (TNF) and interleukin (IL) 1.
- **Janus kinase (JAK) inhibitors**, a class of drugs that block signaling molecules called JAKs to curb cellular processes that lead to the progression of RA.

It is important to work with your doctor to find the right drug, or combination of drugs, to control your disease.

Oral pain-relieving medications. Some medications are designed to relieve pain and some developed for other reasons have been found to relieve pain. Some are available over-the-counter while others require a doctor's prescription. They include:

- **Acetaminophen (*Tylenol*).** An over-the-counter (OTC) analgesic, acetaminophen may be sufficient for mild to moderate osteoarthritis pain. Prescription versions, which combine acetaminophen and a narcotic analgesic, may be used short term to relieve pain after joint surgery.
- **Nonsteroidal anti-inflammatory drugs or NSAIDs.** OTC doses of these drugs, including ibuprofen (*Advil, Motrin IB*) and naproxen sodium (*Aleve*), may be useful for relieving pain. At higher prescription doses they may also relieve inflammation.
- **Duloxetine (*Cymbalta*).** Developed as an antidepressant, duloxetine is also approved for treating chronic pain related to osteoarthritis (OA).
- **Tramadol (*Ultram*).** Available only by prescription, tramadol is an opioid pain reliever prescribed for OA pain not relieved by other medication. Although the risk of addiction and abuse with tramadol is less than that of other opioids, its use is still tightly regulated.

Joint injections are used for acutely painful, inflamed joints.

- **Corticosteroids injections** — strong anti-inflammatory drugs similar to the cortisol made by our bodies — can quickly relieve both pain and inflammation.
- **Hyaluronic acid injections** can relieve painful osteoarthritis. Typically given in a series of injections, hyaluronic acid is a substance that gives joint fluid its natural viscosity. Hyaluronic acid injections are given a week apart in a series of three or four injections.

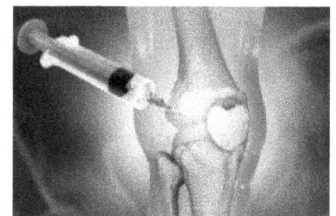

Topical Medications. Topical analgesics are drugs which are applied directly to the skin over the painful joint to relieve pain. They include sprays, creams, ointments and patches, and work by one or a combination of the following ingredients:

- **Capsaicin,** a chemical compound in hot chili peppers, which depletes the nerve cells of substance P, a chemical important for transmitting pain messages.
- **Salicylates**, the same ingredients that relieve pain in aspirin and aspirin-like drugs.
- **Counterirritants**, ingredients such as menthol and camphor, which create a burning and cooling sensation that distract your mind from your pain.
- **Diclofenac,** a prescription NSAID, which may act similarly to oral NSAIDs to relieve pain.

Exercise, Physical Therapies and Devices

Physical Activity. Although joint pain may make activity difficult at first, you'll likely find that once you try it, regular physical activity will actually ease your pain and help your body produce its own natural pain killers — endorphins.

- Physical activity also can increase your strength, stamina, flexibility and range of motion — all of which will help with everyday life. And if you are overweight, staying active can be an important part of a weight-loss plan.
- To avoid causing further pain, choose exercises that are gentle on joints such as walking, stationary cycling, swimming, water aerobics low-impact aerobics or yoga.
- A physical therapist (PT) or occupational therapist (OT) also can help you find and do physical activity that's effective and safe for your specific condition and needs. They can help you adapt the way you move and move your joints — or the environment you live in — so you can safely complete daily tasks like getting in and out of bed, climbing stairs and more.
- To see safe and effective exercises approved by physical therapists, visit the *Arthritis Foundation's Your Exercise Solution.*

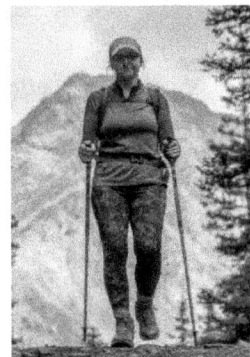

Good Posture. Poor posture can put excessive stress on the joints of the spine, leading to neck and back pain, as well as pain in the extremities. Proper posture, if practiced consistently, can relieve those stresses and associated pain.

- Posture isn't just a matter of standing up straight. A PT or OT can teach you how to use good posture while standing, sitting or moving and even comfortable positioning for relieving joint pain at night.
- A therapist can also help you with specific exercises designed to strengthen specific muscles that help you maintain good posture.

Rest. While it's important to use joints to prevent stiffness, overusing your joints can cause or worsen pain, too. When using a particular joint be sure to take periodic rest breaks. Finding the right balance between activity, rest and down time — that fits your needs — is key to optimizing your joint health and well-being.

Orthotics. Devices such as braces, splints and shoe inserts may be effective in relieving joint pain by shifting weight away from the damaged area of the joint, easing stress on a joint or relieving swelling by compression. A physical or occupational therapist can ensure you have the right orthotic and use it properly.

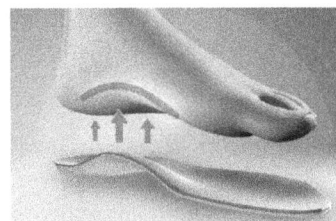

Assistive Devices. Devices are available to help you perform almost any task that causes or exacerbates joint pain, from buttoning blouses to sliding on shoes, to opening jars to reaching items on high shelves. An occupational therapist can help identify devices that would help you and teach you how to use them.

Hot and Cold Therapy.

- Apply heat to aching joints for temporary pain relief. Try a heating pad, hot water bottle, warm compresses, or soak in a hot tub or shower.
- For acutely inflamed and painful joints, try commercial ice packs or a bag of frozen peas or cut vegetables that mold to the shape of your joint and can be used and refrozen multiple times.
- Soaking smaller joints, like hands, feet and elbows, in paraffin wax can also help soothe those painful joints.

Acupuncture. This ancient practice, which involves inserting fine needles at specific points on the body, has been shown to reduce pain in people with some forms of arthritis who have moderate to severe pain despite taking anti-inflammatory or pain medications. However, it may take several weeks before you notice improvement.

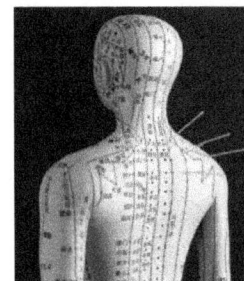

Radiofrequency ablation (RFA). RFA is a procedure in which a doctor inserts a needle guided by X-ray into the painful area of an arthritic joint and then passes a current through the needles to ablate, or burn, the nerve ending to relieve pain.

- RFA is reserved for people for whom less invasive treatments have failed to relieve pain.

Arthritis Surgeries (What to Expect)
Medical News Today

What to expect from arthritis surgery

If arthritis causes serious damage to the joints, a person may require surgery. Arthritis surgery can help fix or replace a damaged joint, reduce pain, and improve the way the joint functions. If standard treatments do not work or the joints become too damaged, arthritis surgery may be necessary.

Benefits of surgery

Arthritis surgery has many benefits, including:

- Reducing joint pain
- Improving joint function
- Preventing further joint damage
- Helping the person reduce their use of anti-inflammatory drugs
- Improving mobility
- Improving daily functioning
- Improving quality of life
- Delaying the need for more intensive surgery, such as a joint replacement

Arthroscopy

- When carrying out an arthroscopy, a surgeon makes a small incision near the joint. They then insert a tiny camera and specialized instruments to fix small tears in the soft tissue within the joint.
- Arthroscopy is a common treatment for arthritis in the knee, hip, shoulder, and other joints.
- A surgeon can also use arthroscopy to remove damaged cartilage and ligaments, as well as broken cartilage pieces that are floating in a joint.
- The Arthritis Foundation does not recommend the use of arthroscopy to treat a type of arthritis called osteoarthritis. It states that a knee arthroscopy rarely relieves pain and that when it does, the relief is often short-lived.

Joint resurfacing

- Joint resurfacing involves replacing part of a joint. The surgeon will remove a damaged part of the joint and replace it with an implant.
- This is an alternative treatment to a total joint replacement.
- During knee joint resurfacing surgery, the surgeon will remove one of the knee's three compartments. They will then replace this with an implant.
- When performing hip joint resurfacing surgery, the surgeon will replace the joint's socket with a metal cup. They may then reshape the damaged hip ball and cap it with a metal, dome-shaped implant.
- This surgery can reduce joint pain and help the joint function correctly.

Osteotomy

- Osteotomy means "cutting of the bone." During this procedure, a surgeon will remove a piece of bone or add a wedge of bone near to a damaged joint.
- A knee osteotomy can help a person who has damage on one side of their knee. The procedure can shift weight away from the damaged side of the joint to help reduce pain and improve knee function.
- A hip osteotomy can correct misalignment of the bones in the joint, known as hip dysplasia, which often occurs in early life.
- According to the Arthritis Foundation, an osteotomy can halt joint damage and delay the need for a joint replacement for 10–15 years.

Synovectomy

- The lining tissue of the joints is called the synovium. Inflammatory arthritis can cause the synovium to become inflamed or grow too much, which can damage the surrounding cartilage and joints.

- During a synovectomy, a surgeon removes most or all of the inflamed synovium. They may carry out this procedure through open surgery or arthroscopy.

A synovectomy can help by:
- Reducing joint pain
- Reducing local tissue and bone damage
- Improving joint function
- Helping the person reduce their use of anti-inflammatory drugs
- However, there is a chance that an open synovectomy will limit the person's range of motion and provide only temporary pain relief.

According to the Arthritis Foundation, arthroscopic synovectomy is a less expensive alternative with fewer complications.

Arthrodesis, or fusion
- If a person has severe joint damage due to osteoarthritis or inflammatory arthritis, they may require arthrodesis or fusion surgery.
- During this procedure, a surgeon will use hardware, such as pins, plates, or rods, to join two or more bones. They may join bones in the ankle, wrist, thumb, finger, or spine to make one continuous joint.
- After surgery, the bones can grow together and lock the joint in place over time.
- This surgery can improve the strength of the joint and reduce joint pain.
- The results of the procedure should last a lifetime, though revisions may be required on occasion.
- The potential downsides are that the fusing of joints can reduce their range of motion and flexibility while also changing their biomechanics. These effects can put added stress on surrounding joints and lead to long-term pain and the development of arthritis in other areas of the body.

Total joint replacement, or total joint arthroplasty
- During a total joint replacement (TJR), a surgeon will remove parts of an arthritic or damaged joint and replace them with a prosthesis.
- The prosthesis can be metal, plastic, or ceramic, and it will replicate the movement of a healthy joint.
- Hip and knee replacements are the most common TJR surgeries. However, a surgeon can also carry out this procedure on other joints, including the ankle, wrist, shoulder, and elbow.

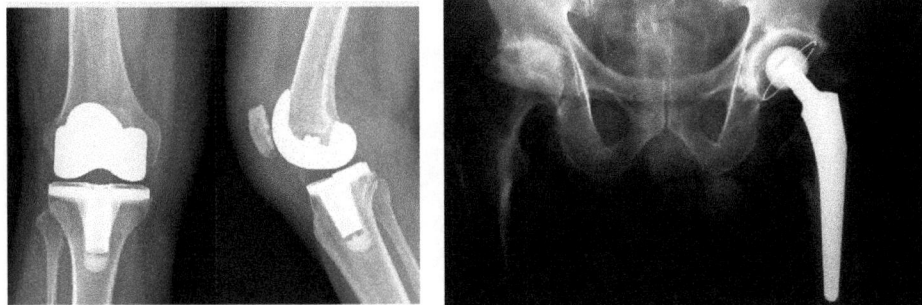

TJR is a safe and effective procedure that can benefit a person by:
- Reducing joint pain
- Improving mobility
- Improving daily functioning
- Boosting the quality of life

Minimally invasive TJR
- A minimally invasive TJR is similar to a regular TJR, but it involves shorter incisions. The surgeon also cuts and reattaches less muscle.
- This procedure still involves cutting and removing bone and adding implants.
- According to the Arthritis Foundation, a minimally invasive TJR results in less pain, less time in the hospital, and a quicker recovery than a regular TJR.

Joint revision
- If a person has an artificial joint or an implant in their joint, it can become worn over time. Most implants can last 15–20 years, but if a person gets one as a young adult, they may eventually require a new one.
- A joint revision is a procedure that aims to remove a damaged implant and replace it with a new one.

This procedure has several benefits, including:
- Relieving pain
- Improving mobility
- Strengthening the joint
- Improving coordination

Revisions are often more complex and less successful than initial joint replacement surgery. This can mean that complete pain relief and a return to full function may not be possible.

Complications
- Arthritis surgery can lead to several complications.
- In some cases, surgery may not be successful, which means that the person may not feel the benefits of the procedure.
- Surgeries that are not successful can limit the range of motion around the affected joint. They may also provide only temporary pain relief.

Other complications of arthritis surgery include:
- Pain
- Infections
- Blood clots
- Injuries to vessels and nerves
- Stiffness in the joint
- Slow healing

Arthritis and Nutrition
The following information is from the Arthritis Foundation by Amy Patural
THE ULTIMATE ARTHRITIS DIET

Is there an arthritis diet?	One of the most common questions people with any form of arthritis have is, "Is there an arthritis diet?" Or more to the point, "What can I eat to help my joints?" The answer, fortunately, is that many foods can help. • Following a diet low in processed foods and saturated fat and rich in fruits, vegetables, fish, nuts, and beans is great for your body. • If this advice looks familiar, it's because these are the principles of the so-called Mediterranean diet, which is frequently touted for its anti-aging, disease-fighting powers.
Benefits	Studies confirm eating these foods can do the following: • Lower blood pressure • Protect against chronic conditions ranging from cancer to stroke • Help arthritis by curbing inflammation • Benefit your joints as well as your heart • Lead to weight loss, which makes a huge difference in managing joint pain.
Should You Avoid Nightshade	• Nightshade vegetables, including eggplant, tomatoes, red bell peppers and potatoes, are disease-fighting powerhouses that boast maximum nutrition for minimal calories. • They also contain solanine, a chemical that has been branded the culprit in arthritis pain. There's no scientific evidence to suggest that nightshades trigger arthritis flares. In fact, some experts believe these vegetables contain a potent nutrient mix that helps inhibit arthritis pain. • However, many people do report significant symptom relief when they avoid nightshade vegetables. So, doctors say, if you notice that your arthritis pain flares after eating them, do a test and try eliminating all nightshade vegetables from your diet for a few weeks to see if it makes a difference.
See Other Charts Below	• Information provided by the **Arthritis Foundation** in chart form based on *The Ultimate Arthritis Diet by Amy Patural* • Anti-inflammatory Diet based on information by **Dr. Weil** • Gluten Free Diet based on research from the **Mayo Clinic, David Perlmutter** and the **Celiac Disease Foundation** • Mediterranean Diet based on information by **Chewfo** and **US News**

The Ultimate Arthritis Diet - Arthritis Foundation

Foods to Eat	How Much	Why	Best Sources
Fish	Health authorities like *The American Heart Association* and *the Academy of Nutrition and Dietetics* recommend three to four ounces of fish, twice a week. Arthritis experts claim more is better.	Some types of fish are good sources of inflammation-fighting omega-3 fatty acids. A study of 727 postmenopausal women, published in the Journal of Nutrition in 2004, found those who had the highest consumption of omega-3s had lower levels of two inflammatory proteins: C-reactive protein (CRP) and interleukin-6. More recently, researchers have shown that taking fish oil supplements helps reduce joint swelling and pain, duration of morning stiffness and disease activity among people who have rheumatoid arthritis (RA).	Salmon Tuna Sardines Herring Anchovies Scallops Other cold-water fish. Supplement. Studies show that taking 600 to 1,000 mg of fish oil daily eases joint stiffness, tenderness, pain and swelling.
Nuts & Seeds	Eat 1.5 ounces of nuts daily (one ounce is about one handful).	Multiple studies confirm the role of nuts in an anti-inflammatory diet," explains José M. Ordovás, PhD, director of nutrition and genomics at the Jean Mayer USDA Human Nutrition Research Center on Aging at Tufts University in Boston. A study published in The American Journal of Clinical Nutrition in 2011 found that over a 15-year period, men and women who consumed the most nuts had a 51 percent lower risk of dying from an inflammatory disease (like RA) compared with those who ate the fewest nuts. Another study, published in the journal Circulation in 2001 found that subjects with lower levels of vitamin B6 – found in most nuts – had higher levels of inflammatory markers. More good news: Nuts are jam-packed with inflammation-fighting monounsaturated fat. And though they're relatively high in fat and calories, studies show noshing on nuts promotes weight loss because their protein, fiber and monounsaturated fats are satiating. "Just keep in mind that more is not always better," says Ordovás.	Walnuts Pine nuts Pistachios Almonds
Fruits & Veggies	Aim for nine or more servings daily (one serving = 1 cup of most veggies or fruit or 2 cups raw leafy greens).	Fruits and vegetables are loaded with antioxidants. These potent chemicals act as the body's natural defense system, helping to neutralize unstable molecules called free radicals that can damage cells. Research has shown that anthocyanins found in cherries and other red and purple fruits like strawberries, raspberries, blueberries, and blackberries have an anti-inflammatory effect. Citrus fruits – like oranges, grapefruits and limes – are rich in vitamin C. Research shows getting the right amount of that vitamin aids in preventing inflammatory arthritis and maintaining healthy joints. Other research suggests eating vitamin K-rich veggies like broccoli, spinach, lettuce, kale and cabbage dramatically reduces inflammatory markers in the blood.	Colorful fruits and veggies – the darker or more brilliant the color, the more antioxidants it has, including Blueberries Cherries Spinach Kale Broccoli

Foods to Eat	How Much	Why	Best Sources
Olive Oil	Two to three tablespoons daily	Olive oil is loaded with heart-healthy fats, as well as oleocanthal, which has properties similar to nonsteroidal, anti-inflammatory drugs. "This compound inhibits activity of COX enzymes, with a pharmacological action similar to ibuprofen," says Ordovás. Inhibiting these enzymes dampens the body's inflammatory processes and reduces pain sensitivity.	Extra virgin olive oil goes through less refining and processing, so it retains more nutrients than standard varieties. Avocado and safflower oils have shown cholesterol-lowering properties. Walnut oil has 10 times the omega-3s that olive oil has.

Beans	About one cup, twice a week (or more)	Beans are loaded with fiber and phytonutrients, which help lower CRP, an indicator of inflammation found in the blood.
		    At high levels, CRP could indicate anything from an infection to RA. In a study published in The *Journal of Food Composition and Analysis* in 2012, scientists analyzed the nutrient content of 10 common bean varieties and identified a host of antioxidant and anti-inflammatory compounds.
		    Beans are also an excellent and inexpensive source of protein, with about 15 grams per cup, which is important for muscle health
			Small red beans
			Red kidney beans
			Pinto beans
			
			These rank among the U.S. Department of Agriculture's top four antioxidant-containing foods (wild blueberries being in the number 2 spot)

Whole Grains	Eat a total of 6 ounces of grains per day; at least 3 of which should come from whole grains. One ounce of whole grain would be equal to ½ cup cooked brown rice or 1 slice of whole-wheat bread.	Whole grains contain plenty of filling fiber – which can help you maintain a healthy weight. Some studies have also shown that fiber and fiber-rich foods can lower blood levels of the inflammatory marker C-reactive protein. ** Some people may need to be careful about which whole grains they eat due to: **Gluten** – a protein found in wheat and other grains that has been linked to inflammation for some people. *See Gluten Free Diet*	Eat foods made with the entire grain kernel, like whole-wheat flour, oatmeal, bulgur, brown rice, and quinoa.

Anti-Inflammatory Diet	Foods to Eat	Foods to avoid	Questionable or Decrease Consumption
(Dr. Weil diet) It is becoming increasingly clear that chronic inflammation is the root cause of many serious illnesses - including heart disease, many cancers, and Alzheimer's disease. We all know inflammation on the surface of the body as local redness, heat, swelling and pain. It is the cornerstone of the body's healing response, bringing more nourishment and more immune activity to a site of injury or infection. But when inflammation persists or serves no purpose, it damages the body and causes illness. Stress, lack of exercise, genetic predisposition, and exposure to toxins (like secondhand tobacco smoke) can all contribute to such chronic inflammation, but dietary choices play a big role as well. Learning how specific foods influence the inflammatory process is the best strategy for containing it and reducing long-term disease risks. *(Dr. Weil)*	Spices and herbs, including turmeric, cinnamon, curry, ginger, garlic, and chili peppers Choose organic fruits and vegetables from all parts of the color spectrum, especially berries, tomatoes, orange and yellow fruits, and dark leafy greens. Mushrooms Winter squashes, and sweet potatoes Cruciferous (cabbage-family) vegetables Beans in general and soybeans in particular. Become familiar with the range of whole-soy foods available and find ones you like. White, green or oolong tea Eat more whole grains such as brown rice and bulgur wheat, in which the grain is intact or in a few large pieces. Extra-virgin olive oil as a main cooking oil. If you want a neutral tasting oil, use expeller-pressed, organic canola oil. Organic, high-oleic, expeller pressed versions of sunflower and safflower oil are also acceptable. Avocados and nuts, especially walnuts, cashews, almonds, and nut butters made from these nuts. For omega-3 fatty acids, eat salmon (preferably fresh or frozen wild or canned sockeye), sardines packed in water or olive oil, herring, and black cod (sablefish, butterfish); omega-3 fortified eggs; hemp seeds and flaxseeds (preferably freshly ground); or take a fish oil supplement (look for products that provide both EPA and DHA, in a convenient daily dosage of two to three grams).	Flour and sugar, especially bread and most packaged snack foods (including chips and pretzels). High fructose corn syrup Butter, cream, high-fat cheese, un-skinned chicken and fatty meats. Products made with palm kernel oil. Safflower and sunflower oils, corn oil, cottonseed oil, and mixed vegetable oils. Strictly avoid margarine, vegetable shortening, and all products listing them as ingredients. Strictly avoid all products made with partially hydrogenated oils of any kind.	Cook pasta al dente and eat it in moderation Animal protein High quality natural cheese and yogurt. Plain dark chocolate in moderation (with a minimum cocoa content of 70 percent). Alcohol (if you must, try red wine)

Gluten Free Diet	Foods to Eat	Foods to Avoid	Questionable or Decrease Consumption	Possible or Other Names to Avoid
A gluten-free diet is a diet that excludes the protein gluten. Gluten is found in grains such as wheat, barley, rye, and a cross between wheat and rye called triticale. *Mayo Clinic* *David Perlmutter* *Celiac Disease Foundation*	Rice Cassava Corn (Maize) Soy Potato Tapioca Beans Sorghum Quinoa Millet Buckwheat Groats *(Also Known as Kasha)* Arrowroot Amaranth Teff Flax Chia Yucca Gluten-Free Oats Nut Flours *(Celiac Disease Foundation)* Beans, seeds and nuts in their natural, unprocessed form Fresh eggs Fresh meats, fish and poultry (not breaded, batter- coated or marinated) Fruits and vegetables Most dairy products *(Mayo Clinic)*	Wheat Wheat germ Rye Barley Bulgur Couscous Farina Graham flour Kamut Matzo Semolina Spelt Triticale Durum flour *(David Perlmutter)*	Malt/Malt Flavoring Soups Commercial Bullion and Broths Cold Cuts, Hot Dogs French Fries (Often Dusted with Flour Before Freezing) Processed Cheese (E.G., Velveeta) Mayonnaise Ketchup Malt Vinegar Soy Sauce And Teriyaki Sauces Salad Dressings Imitation Crab Meat, Bacon, Egg Substitute Tabbouleh Sausage Non-Dairy Creamer Fried Vegetables/Tempura Gravy Marinades Canned Baked Beans Cereals Commercially Prepared Chocolate Milk Breaded Foods Fruit Fillings and Puddings Ice Cream Root Beer Energy Bars, Trail Mix Syrups Seitan Wheatgrass Instant Hot Drinks Flavored Coffees and Teas Blue Cheeses Vodka, Wine Coolers Meatballs, Meatloaf Communion Wafers Veggie Burgers Roasted Nuts Beer Oats or Oat Bran (Unless Certified Gf) *(David Perlmutter)*	Avena sativa Cyclodextrin Dextrin Fermented grain extract Hordeum distichon Hordeum vulgare Hydrolysate Hydrolyzed malt extract Hydrolyzed vegetable protein Maltodextrin Phytosphingosine extract Samino peptide complex Secale cereale Triticum aestivum Triticum vulgare Tocopherol/Vit. E Yeast extract Natural flavoring Brown rice syrup Modified food starch Hydrolyzed vegetable protein (HVP) Hydrolyzed Soy protein Caramel color (frequently made from barley) *(David Perlmutter)*

Mediterranean Diet	Foods to Eat	Foods to avoid	Questionable or Decrease Consumption
Harvard School of Public Health, Oldways, a nonprofit food think tank in Boston, developed a consumer-friendly Mediterranean diet pyramid that emphasizes fruits, veggies, whole grains, beans, nuts, legumes, olive oil and flavorful herbs and spices; eating fish and seafood at least a couple of times a week; enjoying poultry, eggs, cheese, and yogurt in moderation; and saving sweets and red meat for special occasions. *Chewfo* *US News*	Fruits Vegetables Whole Grains Olive oil Beans Nuts Legumes Seeds Herbs Spices Seafood	Sugar-sweetened beverages Added sugar Processed meat Refined grains Refined oils Highly processed foods Fast Foods	Red Meat Salt Cheese and yogurt Milk Crème Poultry Eggs Sweeteners, such as honey Wine

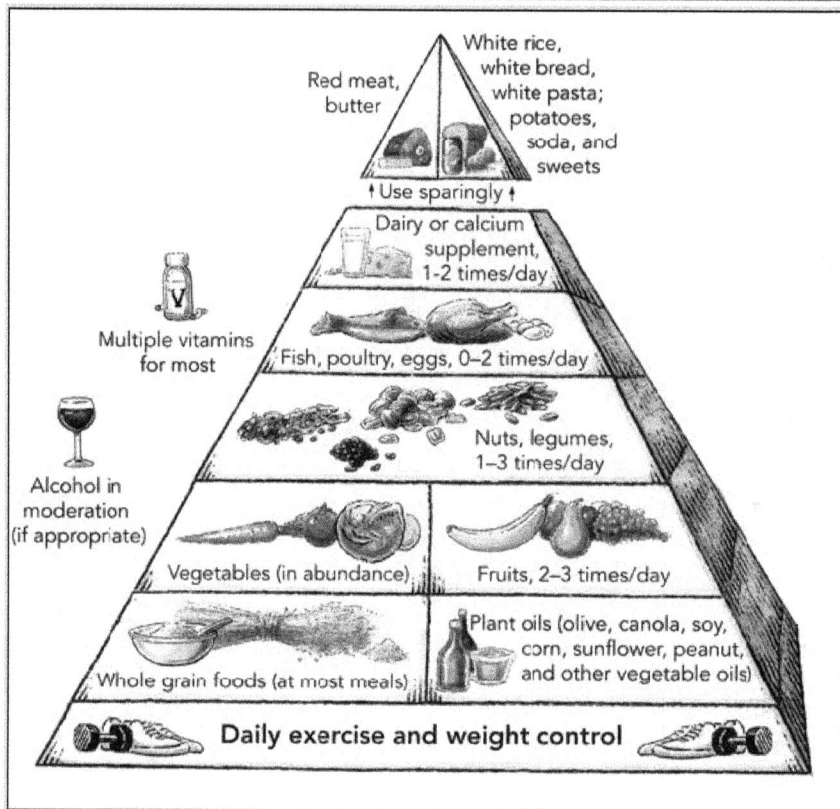

Arthritis & Osteoporosis References

ACE – Fitness Professionals Guide to Training Clients with Osteoarthritis

American College of Sports Medicine - *(ACSM) https://www.acsm.org/*

Arthritis Foundation - *www.arthritis.org/living-with-arthritis/exercise/*

Arthritis Foundation: *Finding the Best Joint Pain Relief for You: 24 Treatment Options* by *Mary Anne Dunkin*: **Oral, Injected and Topical Medications** and **Exercise, Physical Therapies and Devices** - *https://www.arthritis.org/health-wellness/healthy-living/managing-pain/pain-relief-solutions/finding-the-best-joint-pain-relief*

Arthritis Foundation: *The Ultimate Arthritis Diet* by *Amy Patural* - *www.arthritis.org/living-with-arthritis/arthritis-diet/anti-inflammatory/the-arthritis-diet.php*

Association of Rheumatology Health Professionals (Now the Rheumatologist) (ARHP) - *https://www.the-rheumatologist.org/article/association-of-rheumatology-professionals-new-name-but-the-commitment-remains-the-same/*

CDC.gov - *cdc.gov/nccdphp/dnpa/physical/growing_stronger/*

Celiac Disease Foundation - *celiac.org/live-gluten-free/glutenfreediet/food-options/#B3q0UllhdleaKFky.99*

Chewfo - *www.chewfo.com/diets/the-mediterranean-diet-cookbook-by-rockridge-press-2013-food-list-what-to-eat-and-foods-to- avoid/*

David Perlmutter - *www.drperlmutter.com/eat/foods-that-contain-gluten/*

Dr. Weil - *www.drweil.com/drw/u/ART02012/anti-inflammatory-diet*

Mayo Clinic - *www.mayoclinic.org/healthy-lifestyle/nutrition-and-healthy-eating/in-depth/gluten-free-diet/art-20048530*

Medical News Today: *What to expect from arthritis surgery* - Medically reviewed by Nancy Carteron, M.D., FACR — Written by Adam Rowden on March 3, 2022 - *https://www.medicalnewstoday.com/articles/arthritis-surgery*

MedicineNet.com

National Institute of Arthritis and Musculoskeletal and Skin Diseases (NISM) - *https://www.nih.gov/about-nih/what-we-do/nih-almanac/national-institute-arthritis-musculoskeletal-skin-diseases-niams*

National Osteoporosis Foundation – *(Now the Bone Health and Osteoporosis Foundation (BHOF))* - *https://www.bonehealthandosteoporosis.org/news/national-osteoporosis-foundation-is-now-bone-health-and-osteoporosis-foundation/*

NIA Publications - *www.niapublications.org/exercisebook/chapter4_strength.htm*

Prevention
https://www.prevention.com/health/dietlowersalzheimersrisk

US News - *https://health.usnews.com/best-diet/mediterranean-diet*

WebMD.com

Safety First

- Benefits / Before Starting a Routine
- Averages, Body Temperature
- Respiration, Blood Pressure, Heart Rate
- How to Monitor Intensity of Heart Rate
- Temperature – Heat and Cold
- Dehydration; Altitude

Components of a Conditioning Program

- Warm up/cool down
- Duration, Frequency, Intensity & Movement Patterns
- Breathing – Diaphragmatic, Pursed lip and with Exercise
- Equipment That May be Needed

Self-Tests:

- Prior to starting program

Exercise Worksheets:

- Exercises below with:
  - Exercise name and number for section
  - Reps, Sets, How many times a day and how long a stretch should be held (Ex. 20 seconds)

EXERCISE Flexibility (Stretching)	EXERCISE NUMBER	PAGE	REPS	SETS	X DAY	HOLD
PRAYER STRETCH and LATERAL	53					

Exercises:

- Myofascial release
- Flexibility / Stretches / ROM
- Core / Abdominal
- Strengthening - Upper and Lower Extremity
- Balance > Lower Extremity Standing Exercises
- Agility
- Endurance/Aerobic Capacity
- Calories
- Worksheet with room for notes under each section

EXERCISE Core / Stability / Balance	EXERCISE NUMBER	NOTES
PRONE BALL	27	

References

PHYSICAL AND PSYCHOLOGICAL BENEFITS OF KEEPING PHYSICALLY FIT

- Contributes positively to maintaining a healthy weight, building and maintaining healthy bone density, muscle strength, joint mobility, reducing surgical risks, and strengthening the immune system.
- Helps to prevent or treat serious and life-threatening chronic conditions such as high blood pressure, obesity, heart disease, Type 2 diabetes, insomnia, and depression.
- Endurance exercise before meals lowers blood glucose more than the same exercise after meals.
- It also improves mental health, helps prevent depression, helps to promote or maintain positive self-esteem, and can even augment an individual's sex appeal or body image.

(Physical Exercise - Wikipedia)

Before starting a routine here are some factors to consider

AGE	Men over 45 and women over 55 should have medical evaluation before starting a vigorous exercise program. If you will be participating in low to moderate exercise, it is suggested that those with, or have signs and symptoms of cardiopulmonary disease, set up a medical evaluation.
MEDICAL AND PHYSICAL CONDITION	It is very important for you to be aware of any medical or physical problems that may impede your performance. **If you have any of the following issues, please see a medical doctor and/or physical therapist to address issues before starting an exercise program:** <ul><li>Cardiac issues</li><li>Pulmonary issues</li><li>Arthritis</li><li>Joint pain</li><li>Back pain</li><li>Diabetes</li><li>Acute or Chronic issues, such as, but not limited to, Parkinson's, Stroke, Autoimmune Diseases, Metabolic Disease or Orthopedic disorders/joint replacements.</li></ul>

VITAL SIGN AVERAGES

Adult (resting)	
Body Temperature	98.6 Fahrenheit under tongue.
Respiration	12-20 breaths per minute

Blood Pressure
 	
Systolic/Diastolic
	120/80.
	Systolic is when the heart pumps blood to the body / Diastolic is blood that remains in arteries when the heart relaxes.
	Pre-hypertension: 120-139/80-89.
	Hypertension:
	     Stage I 140-159/90-99
	     Stage II over 160/100

Resting pulse	**Men**: 70 beats per minute. **Women:** 75 beats per minute.

HOW to MONITOR EXERCISE INTENSITY

Ways to monitor heart rate (HR):

Talk Test Method	This is a simple, subjective method for the beginner to determine your comfort zone while exercising. Are you able to breathe and talk comfortably throughout the workout without gasping for air? If not, reduce your activity level, catch your breath, and resume at a slower pace.
Heart Rate monitor or Watch	This is a device you wear on your wrist or chest, which allows you to measure your heart rate in real time. These devices range in price at about $50.00 for just a basic HR monitor or higher with other bells and whistles. Some of the popular manufacturers are Fitbit, Apple Watch, Garmin and Samsung Galaxy among others. (See *Target Heart Rate*)
Rate of Perceived Exertion	This method was designed by Dr. Gunnar Borg and is often called the Borg Scale (revised). It rates what you feel your level of exertion is from a scale of 1-10, one being at rest and ten at maximal exertion. A rate of 5-7 is recommended, somewhere between somewhat hard and very hard. Like the talk test method, this is subjective and should be used with HR monitoring.
Training Heart Rate	Measuring Heart Rate: Place your first and second finger over the pulse site and gently apply pressure. Palpate the number of beats for a full minute or 30 sec x 2, 15 sec x 4 or 6 sec x 10. If you have in irregular heartbeat, it is suggested counting the full 60 seconds. Do not use the thumb, as this has its own pulse.
	Take your pulse after you've been exercising for at least five minutes. An easy way to check your pulse without interrupting your workout too much is to take a quick 6-second count and then multiply that number by 10 to get your heart rate in beats per minute (BPM). Make sure your pulse is within your target heart rate zone (*see below*). You can then increase or decrease your intensity based on your heart rate. You can also wear a heart rate monitor. Radial: Wrist following line from base of thumb. Carotid: Side of larynx.
Target heart rate range (THR)	**Beginner or low fitness level**: 50-60% **Intermediate or average fitness level:** 60-70% **Advanced or high fitness level:** 75-85%
Percent of maximal heart rate	220 - Age = predicted maximum heart rate (HR). To get the desired exercise intensity, multiply the predicted maximal HR by the percentage. For example, a woman who is 40 years old of Intermediate fitness level would use the following equation at a 70% target heart rate: 220 – 40 (age) =180 predicted maximal HR. 180 x 0.70 (THR) = 126 BPM - desired exercise HR.
Karvonen Formula	Percentage of Heart-rate reserve. This formula factors in the resting HR as well, which will make the target heart rate higher than just the percentage of maximal heart rate. To figure this out, take the predicted maximal heart rate as above with a resting HR prior to exercise. Maximal HR – resting heart rate (RHR) = heart rate reserve; multiply by intensity + RHR + Target HR. See example under Percentage of maximal HR. Rest heart rate = 80. 220 – 40 (age) =180 (as above) – 80 (RHR) = 100 x 0.70 (THR) = 70 + 80 = 150 Target HR.

TEMPERATURE – HEAT and COLD

HEAT

Avoid exercise in the hottest part of the day, as well as in humid weather. People need to sweat to regulate internal body temperature and must evaporate to dissipate heat. During hot, humid weather, sweat cannot evaporate, and therefore cannot cool the body down. It is also important to drink plenty of cool water during exercise, about 7-10 oz. every 10-20 minutes during exercise (see *Dehydration*).

Heat cramps:	• Severe cramps that begin in hands, feet or calves • Hard, tense muscles
Heat exhaustion: Requires immediate medical attention, although not usually life threatening	• Fatigue • Nausea • Headache • Excessive thirst • Muscle aches and cramps • Confusion or anxiety • Weakness • Severe sweats that can be accompanied by cold, clammy skin • Slow heartbeat (decreased pulse rate) • Dizziness or fainting • Agitation
Heat Stroke: Can occur suddenly, with or without warning from heat exhaustion. Obtain immediate medical attention, as this can be *fatal*	• Nausea and vomiting • Headache • Increased body temperature, but DECREASED sweating. • Hot, flushed, DRY skin • Dizziness • Fatigue • Rapid heart rate • Shortness of breath • Decreased urination or may have blood in the urine. • Confusion or loss of consciousness • Convulsions

COLD

It is just as important to drink plenty of water when exercising in the cold weather secondary to increased urine production.   Be sure to dress in layers to help self-regulate body temperature. This simply involves taking off or putting back on clothing as dictated by the changing weather conditions. Choose clothing that will keep moisture out and away from the skin, such as Gortex® brand. Clothing that stays wet because of sweat will decrease your body temperature.

Hypothermia-Mild: A body temperature that is below normal. People with hypothermia are usually not aware of their condition due to confusion or being overly focused on their current activity. Hypothermia may or may not include shivering in the early stages	• Confusion • Lack of coordination • Fatigue • Nausea or vomiting • Dizziness
Hypothermia	• Shivering • Slurred speech • Mumbling • Clumsiness • Difficulty speaking • Stumbling • Poor decision making • Drowsiness • Weak pulse • Shallow breathing • Progressive loss of consciousness

DEHYDRATION

Excessive loss of body fluid (which can include water and solutes, usually sodium or electrolytes). It is also important to drink plenty of cool water during exercise, about 7-10 oz. every 10-20 minutes during exercise. During exercise, sports drinks may be necessary to keep an electrolyte balance as well.

Dehydration-Mild: About 2% of water depletion	• Thirst • Decreased urine volume • Abnormally dark urine • Unexplained tiredness • Irritability • Lack of tears when crying • Headache • Dry mouth • Dizziness when standing due to orthostatic hypotension • May cause insomnia.
Moderate: About 5% -6%of water depletion	• Grogginess or sleepiness • Headache • Nausea • May feel tingling in limbs (parenthesis)
Severe: About 10% -15% of water depletion	• Muscles may become spastic • Skin may shrivel and wrinkle (decreased skin turgor) • Vision may dim • Urination will be greatly reduced and may become painful • Delirium may begin.
Over 15% of water depletion	• Usually, fatal.

COMPONENTS OF A CONDITIONING PROGRAM

WARM UP and COOL DOWN

Warming up and cooling down are very important parts of the exercise routine. There are physical and psychological benefits to both these components that can be as simple as a slow walk before and after your exercise program.

Benefits of warming up	Benefits of cooling down
• Increases the temperature in the muscles, which increases the speed of contraction and relaxation. • Reduces premature lactic acid build up and fatigue during high level exercises. • Increases speed of nerve impulse conduction. • Increases elasticity of connective tissues • Increases muscle metabolism and oxygen consumption that enhances aerobic performance. • Alert for potential muscle injury that may arise during higher intensities. • Increases endorphins. • Allows the heart rate to get to a workable rate for beginning exercise. • Increases production of synovial fluid located between the joints to reduce friction. • Psychological warm up to mentally focus on training and competition.	• Prevents venous blood pooling at the extremities, which reduces chance of dizziness or fainting. • Reduces the potential for Delayed Onset Muscle Soreness (DOMS). • Aids in removing waste products in muscles, such as lactic acid. • Reduces the level of adrenaline and other exercise hormones in the blood to lower the chance of post-exercise disturbances in cardiac rhythm. • Allows the heart to return back safely to resting rate.

Start out every routine with a warmup first. Here are some suggestions

- Walking or outside
- Running up and down some stairs
- Jumping jacks
- Running in place
- Dynamic stretching

Equipment

- Treadmill
- Stationary or Recumbent bike
- Stair climber or Elliptical
- Mini trampoline

Duration, Frequency, Intensity and Movement Patterns

Intensity: How *much* mental and physical *effort* it takes to sustain an activity.	This can be done using the target heart rate range THR (optimum exercise intensity levels through beats per minute, talk test or rate of perceived exertion.
Duration: How *long* the training lasts.	The higher the intensity, the shorter the duration. The American College of Sports Medicine guidelines recommends all healthy adults aged 18–65 yr should participate in moderate intensity aerobic physical activity for a minimum of 30 min on five days per week, or vigorous intensity aerobic activity for a minimum of 20 min on three days per week.
Frequency: How *often* the training occurs.	Training should be performed at least every other day or three days a week. Cardiac/aerobic conditioning can be done daily, although you may want to vary exercises. Regarding strength training, it is important to give each muscle group 48 hours to recover. Alternate upper and lower body with isolated abdomen/core exercises every other day. For those working out several days a week, find a schedule that works for you as long as you give each muscle group 48 hours of recovery time.

Movement Patterns and Examples
 	
Basic movements that help to increase overall body strengthening
	• Bend and Lift: Squats, Dead Lifts and Leg presses
	   o Picking up item off floor
	• Single Leg: Step ups, Single leg stance, Lunges
	   o Walking up steps
	• Push: Shoulder press, Bench press, Push up
	   o Pushing Shopping cart or Lawn mower
	• Pull: Lat pull downs, Seated rows
	   o Vacuuming, Raking
	• Rotational
	   o Shoveling snow

Diaphragmatic Breathing

- Lie either on your back with your knees bent or sit up
- Inhale through your nose; as you do so, allow your stomach to rise. Limit movement in your chest. Attempt to push your bottom ribs out to the side as you breathe in.
- Exhale through your mouth; as you do so, allow your stomach to fall. Limit movement in your chest.
- Repeat for at least 10 cycles.

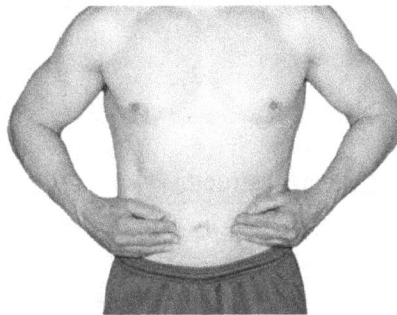

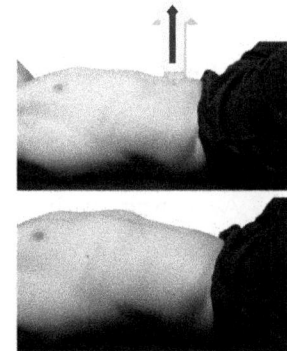

Pursed Lip Breathing

(PLB) is a breathing technique that consists of inhaling through the nose with the mouth closed and then exhaling through tightly pressed (pursed) lips. This technique is frequently in those with cardiac or respiratory issues. *"Smell the Roses then Blow Out the Candle".*

Breathing with Exercise

Exhale on the exertion. For example, exhale when you are lying on your back and pushing a weight up or when bending your arm doing a bicep curl,. Inhale as you bring the weight slowly to your chest or when you straighten your arm with a bicep curl..

ANATOMY

ANATOMICAL POSITIONS and PLANES

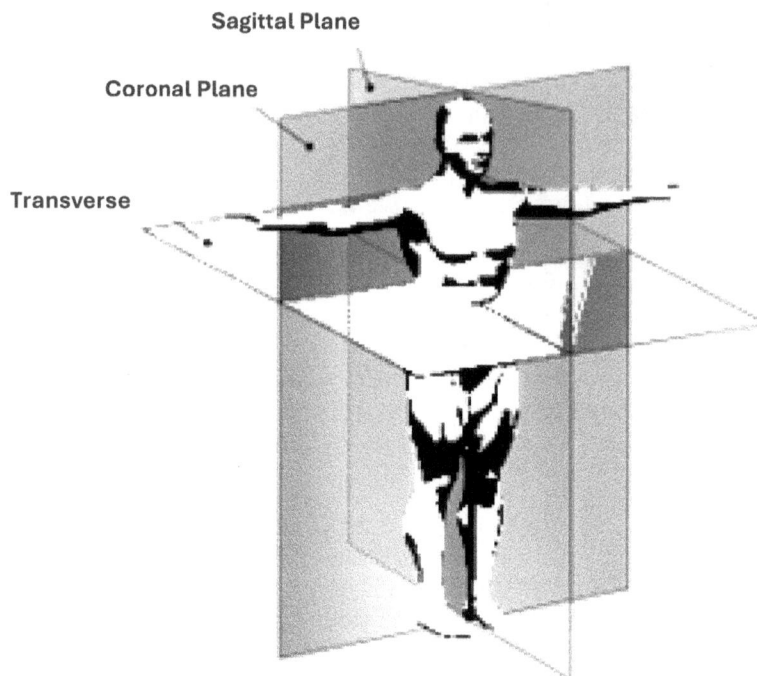

Anterior – Towards the front of the body.

Posterior – Towards the back of the body.

Distal – Away from the body or any point of reference, or from the point of attachment or origin.

Proximal – Closer to the body or any point of reference, or to the point of attachment or origin.

Medial – Situated towards the midline of the body.

Lateral – Position farther from the midline of the body.

Inferior – Away from the head or lower surface of a structure.

Superior – Towards the head or situated above.

Transverse /Axial / Horizontal plane is parallel to the ground, which separates the superior from the inferior or the head from the feet.

Coronal / Frontal/Frontal plane is perpendicular to the ground, which separates the anterior from the posterior or the front from the back

Sagittal / Lateral plane is a Y-Z plane, perpendicular to the ground, which separates left from right.

Upper Extremity (UE): Shoulders, Chest, Arms, Hands, etc

Lower Extremity (LE): Hips, Legs, Ankle Foot , etc

ANATOMICAL DIRECTIONS

Range of Motion (ROM): The distance and direction a joint can move between the flexed and extended position (*see flexion and extension below*). This can also be the act of attempting to increase the distance through therapeutic exercise and/or stretching for physiological gain.

Flexion - Bending movement that decreases the angle between two parts. Bending the knee or elbow are examples of flexion. Flexion of the hip or shoulder moves the limb forward (towards the front of the body).

Extension - The opposite of flexion; a straightening movement that increases the angle between body parts. The knees are extended when standing up. When straightening the arm, the elbow is extended. Extension of the hip or shoulder moves the limb backward (towards the back of the body).

Hyperextension – Extending the joint beyond extension.

Abduction - A lateral movement that pulls a structure or part away from the midline of the body. Raising the arms to the sides is an example of abduction.

Adduction - A medial movement that pulls a structure or part towards the midline of the body, or towards the midline of a limb. Dropping the arms to the sides, or bringing the knees together, are examples of adduction.

Internal rotation (or *medial rotation*). Inward rotary movement around the axis of the bone. Internal rotation of the shoulder or hip would point the toes or the flexed forearm inwards (towards the midline).

External rotation (or *lateral rotation*). External rotary movement around the axis of the bone. It would turn the toes or the flexed forearm outwards (away from the midline).

Elevation - Movement in a superior direction. Shrugging or bringing the shoulders up is an example of elevation.

Depression - Movement in an inferior direction, the opposite of elevation. Pushing the shoulders down is an example of depression.

Pronation - Internal rotation the hand or foot to face downward or posterior. Pronating the foot is a combination of eversion and abduction.

Supination - External rotation of the hand or foot to face upward or anterior. Raising the inside or medial margin of the foot.

Dorsiflexion – Movement at the ankle of the foot superiorly towards the shin. The up position of tapping the foot.

Plantarflexion – Movement at the ankle of the foot inferiorly away from the shin. Pointing the foot downward.

Eversion – Moving the sole of the foot away from the median plane or outward.

Inversion - Moving the sole of the foot towards the median plane or inward.

Ipsilateral – Same side of the body

Contralateral – Opposite side of the body

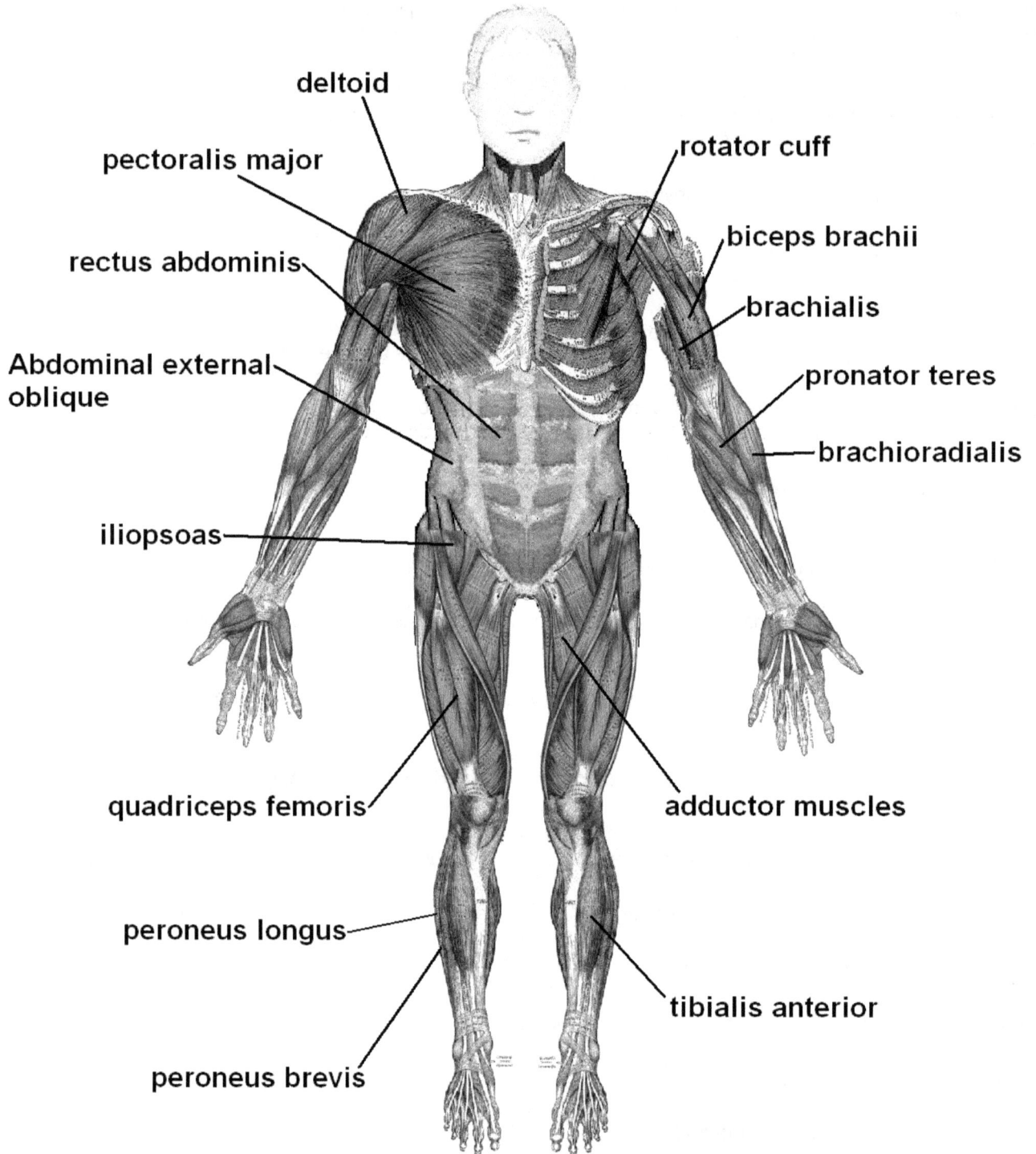

MUSCLES

Grey's Anatomy

ANTERIOR

deltoid

pectoralis major

rectus abdominis

Abdominal external oblique

iliopsoas

quadriceps femoris

peroneus longus

peroneus brevis

rotator cuff

biceps brachii

brachialis

pronator teres

brachioradialis

adductor muscles

tibialis anterior

Muscle Name (AKA)	Joint Action
Pectoralis major	Shoulder flexion, adduction, internal rotation
Deltoid (anterior)	Shoulder abduction, flexion, internal rotation
Rotator cuff (SITS) Supraspinatus Infraspinatus Teres minor Subscapularis	Shoulder: Supraspinatus: Abduction Infraspinatus: External rotation Teres minor: External rotation Subscapularis: Internal rotation
Biceps brachii	Elbow flexion; Forearm supination
Brachialis	Elbow flexion
Pronator teres	Elbow flexion; Forearm pronation
Brachioradialis	Elbow flexion
Tensor fasciae latae	Hip flexion, medial rotation & abduction
Gracilis*	Hip adduction & internal rotation;Knee flexion & internal rotation
Adductor muscles Adductor magnus, longus & brevis	Hip adduction
Tibialis anterior	Ankle dorsiflexion; foot inversion
Peroneus brevis	Ankle plantarflexion; Foot eversion
Peroneus longus	Ankle plantarflexion; Foot eversion
Rectus femoris (quadriceps femoris)	Hip extension (esp. when knee is extended); Knee flexion
Vastus medialis	Knee extension (esp. when hip is flexed)
Vastus lateralis	Knee extension (esp. when hip is flexed)
Sartorius	Hip flexion & external rotation; Knee flexion & internal rotation
Pectineus	Hip adduction
Iliopsoas, Psosas, Iliacus	Hip flexion & external rotation
Abdominal external oblique	Trunk lateral flexion
Rectus abdominis	Trunk flexion & lateral flexion
Abdominal internal oblique	Trunk lateral flexion

MUSCLES

Grey's Anatomy

POSTERIOR

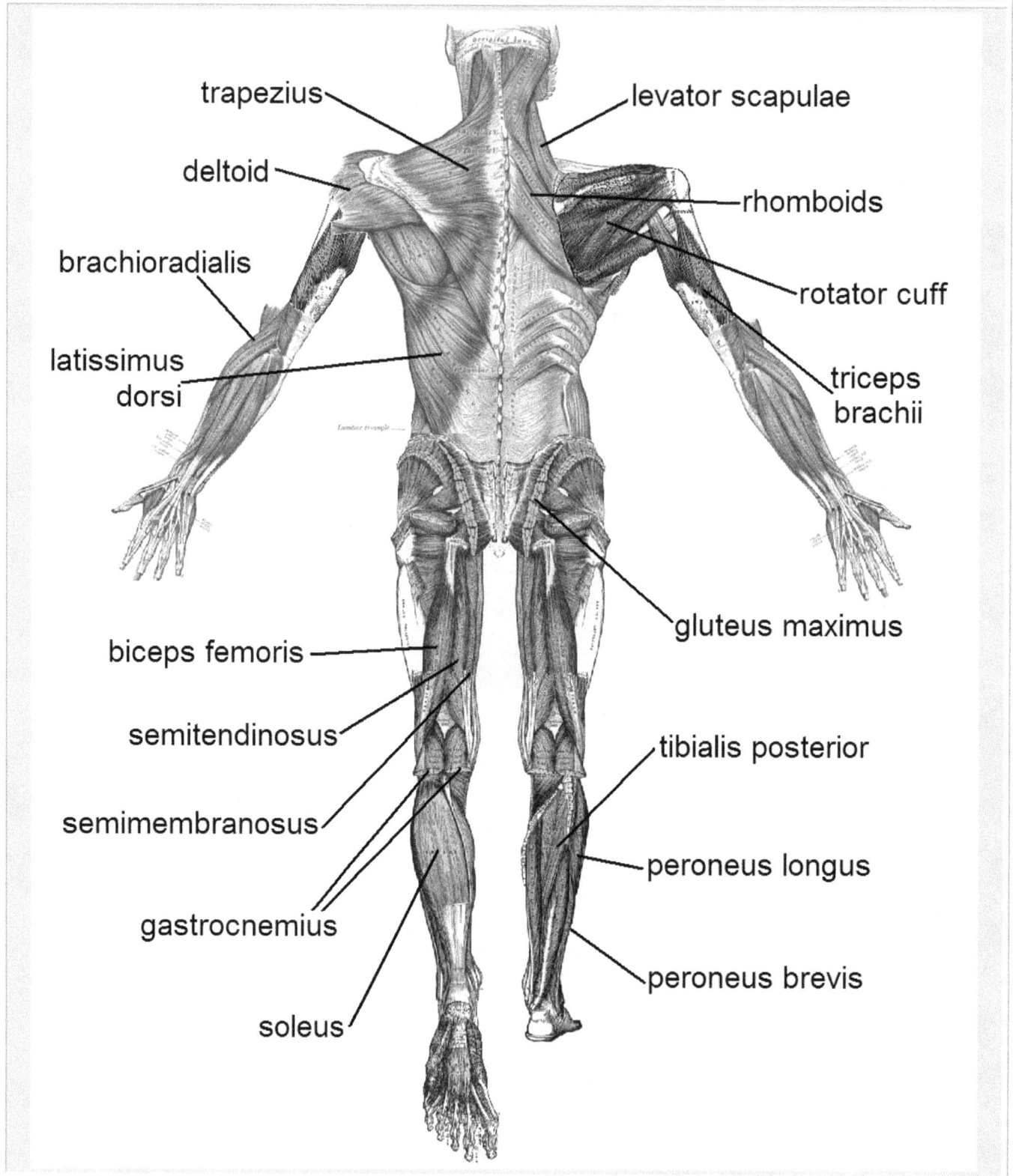

trapezius

levator scapulae

deltoid

rhomboids

brachioradialis

rotator cuff

latissimus
dorsi

triceps
brachii

gluteus maximus

biceps femoris

semitendinosus

tibialis posterior

semimembranosus

peroneus longus

gastrocnemius

peroneus brevis

soleus

Muscle Name (AKA)	Joint Action
Deltoid (posterior)	Shoulder abduction, extension, external rotation
Trapezius	Scapula or Shoulder girdle:, Upper traps: Scapula elevation. Middle traps: Scapula adduction. Lower traps: Scapula depression
Levator scapulae	Scapula elevation
Rhomboids	Scapula adduction & elevation
Triceps brachii	Elbow extension
Gluteus medius	Hip abduction
Gluteus maximus	Hip extension & external rotation
Tibialis, posterior	Inversion, stabilization, assists with plantarflexion
Soleus	Ankle plantarflexion
Gastrocnemius	Knee flexion; Ankle plantarflexion
Semimembranosus	Hip extension & internal rotation; Knee flexion & internal rotation
Semitendinosus	Hip extension & internal rotation; Knee flexion & internal rotation
Biceps femoris (long head)	Hip extension & internal rotation; Knee flexion & external rotation
Latissimus dorsi	Shoulder extension, adduction, internal rotation
Erector spinae, Longissimus, Spinalis, Iliocostalis	Trunk extension, hyperextension & lateral flexion Deep muscle that originate in the posterior iliac crest & sacrum running up the spine and inserts in the transverse process of ribs
Pes anserine, Gracilis, Sartorius, Semimembranosus, Semitendinosus	Internal rotation of tibia when knee is flexed

SKELETON

ANTERIOR (FRONT)

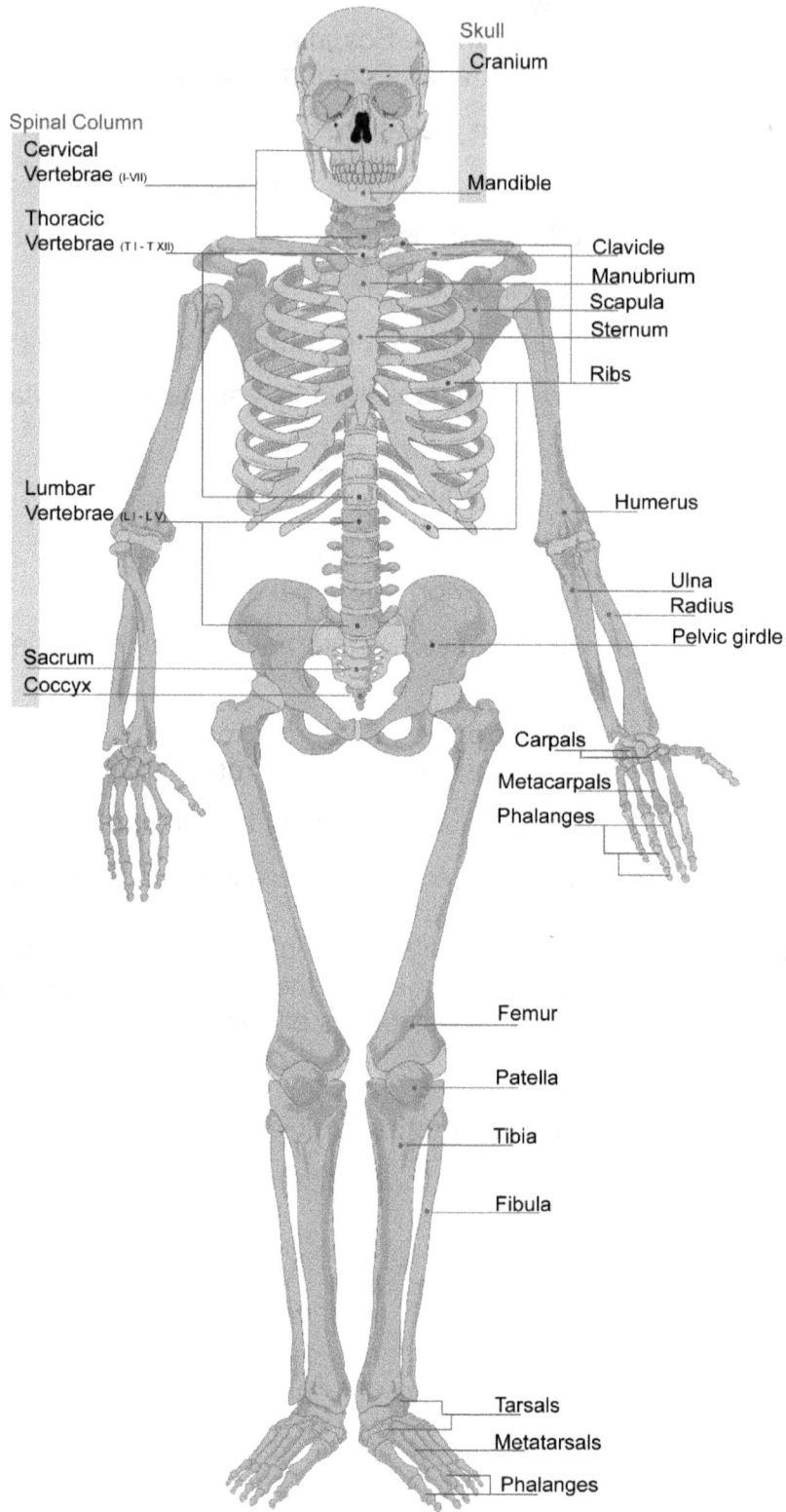

Skull
Cranium

Spinal Column
Cervical
Vertebrae (I-VII)

Mandible

Thoracic
Vertebrae (T I - T XII)

Clavicle
Manubrium
Scapula
Sternum

Ribs

Humerus

Lumbar
Vertebrae (L I - L V)

Ulna
Radius
Pelvic girdle

Sacrum
Coccyx

Carpals
Metacarpals
Phalanges

Femur

Patella

Tibia

Fibula

Tarsals
Metatarsals
Phalanges

SKELETON

POSTERIOR (BACK)

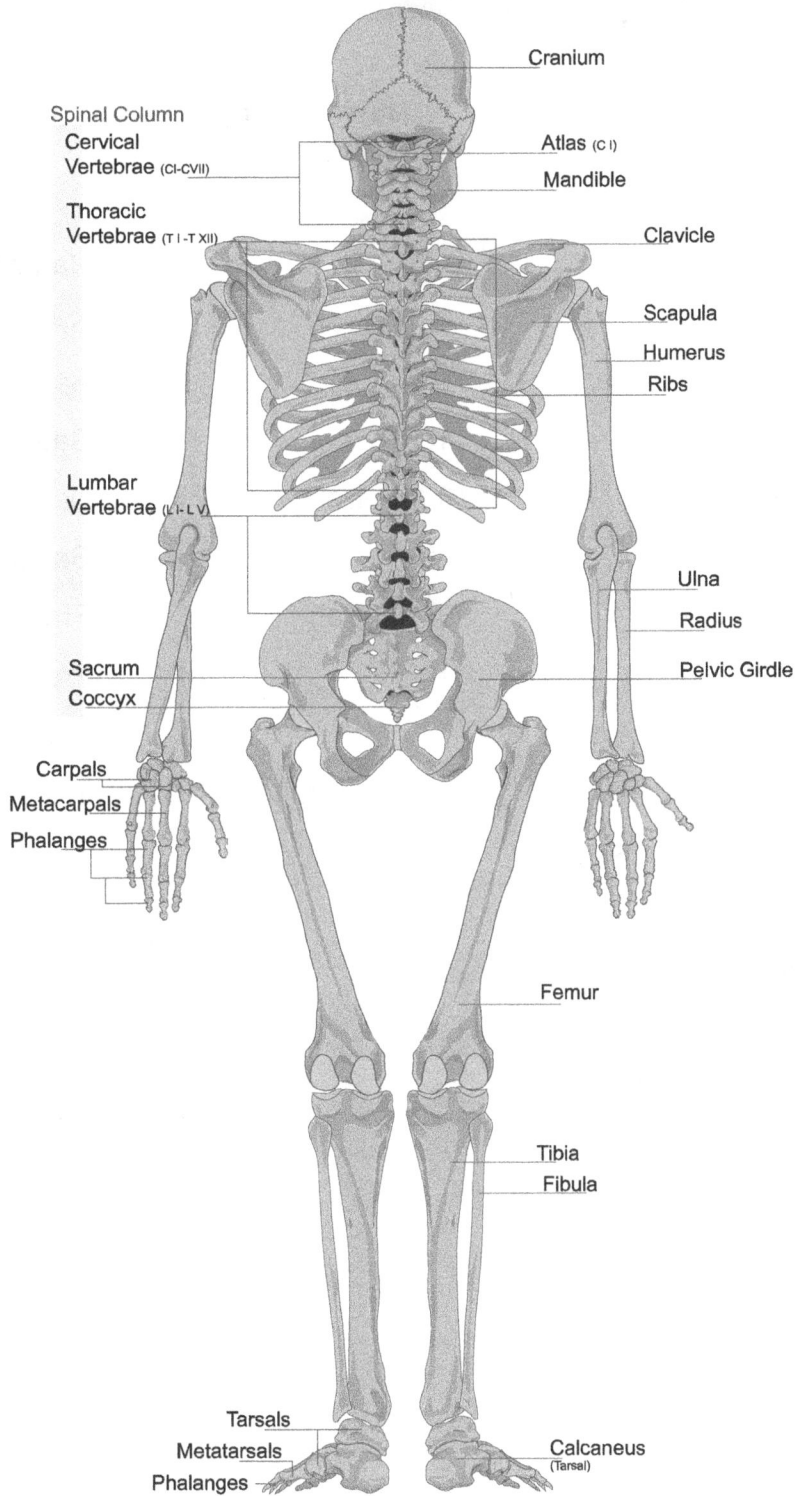

Cranium

Spinal Column
Cervical
Vertebrae (CI-CVII)

Atlas (C I)
Mandible

Thoracic
Vertebrae (T I -T XII)

Clavicle

Scapula
Humerus
Ribs

Lumbar
Vertebrae (LI-LV)

Ulna
Radius

Sacrum
Coccyx

Pelvic Girdle

Carpals
Metacarpals
Phalanges

Femur

Tibia
Fibula

Tarsals
Metatarsals
Phalanges

Calcaneus
(Tarsal)

Average Joint Range of Motion

Anatomical Positions – Upper Extremity

Joint UPPER EXTREMITY	Movement	Normal Range of Motion (degrees)	Plane
Elbow	Flexion	150	Sagittal
	Extension	0 (neutral)	Sagittal
	Hyperextension	< 10	Sagittal
Shoulder	Flexion	180	Sagittal
	Extension	0 (neutral)	Sagittal
	Hyperextension	60	Sagittal
	Adduction (Add)	0 (neutral)	Frontal
	Abduction (Abd)	180	Frontal
	Horizontal Add/Flexion	130	Transverse
	Horizontal Abd	0 (to neutral)	Transverse
	Horizontal Extension	45	Transverse
	Internal rotation	70	Sagittal
	External rotation	90	Sagittal
Radioulnar	Pronation	90	Transverse
	Supination	90	Transverse

Average Joint Range of Motion

Anatomical Positions – Lower Extremity

Joint LOWER EXTREMITY	Movement	Normal Range of Motion (degrees)	Plane
Knee	Flexion	135	Sagittal
	Extension	0 (neutral)	Sagittal
	Hyperextension	10	Sagittal
Hip	Flexion	120	Sagittal
	Extension	0 (neutral)	Sagittal
	Hyperextension	< 20	Sagittal
	Adduction (Add)	0 (neutral)	Frontal
	Abduction (Abd)	50	Frontal
	Internal rotation	40	Transverse
	External rotation	50	Transverse
Ankle	Dorsiflexion	20	Sagittal
	Plantarflexion	50	Sagittal

EQUIPMENT used in this Book.

Don't buy a lot of equipment before knowing what your goals are.

Stability / Exercise Ball Bosu

These can replace an exercise bench if you do not have the space. It is also used for many of the core strengthening exercises

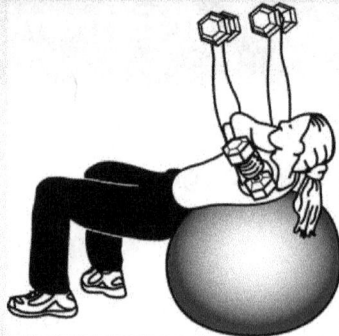

Should be inflated so that when you sit on it you are at a 90-degree angle.

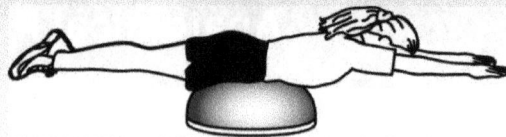

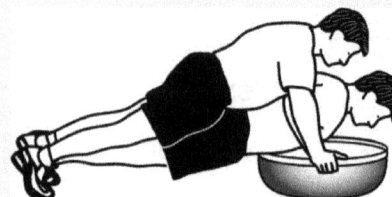

Dumbbells

Kettle Bell (optional)

Dowel with/without weight

These will be needed for your strength exercises. See *Strengthening* section on for resistance.

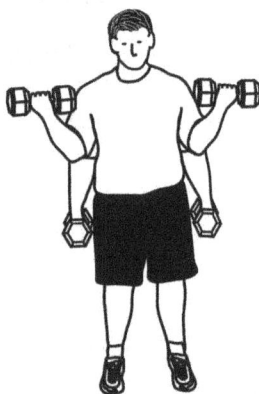

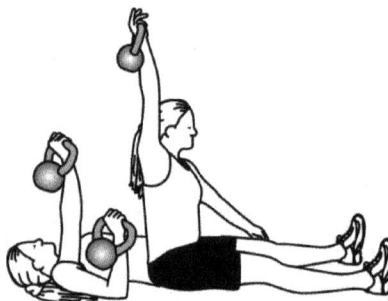

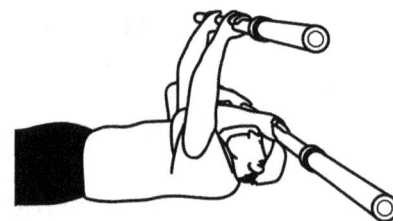

Resistance bands

In different weights/ resistance.

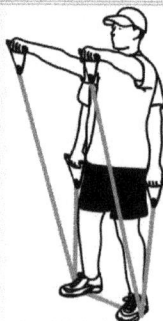

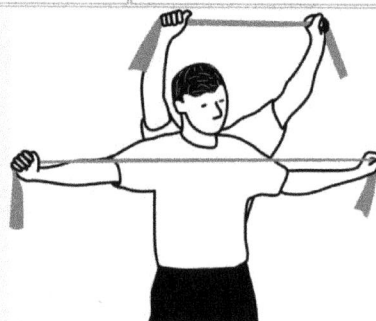

Agility Equipment

Cone hurdles, Speed hurdles, Agility ladder/rings/poles, Bosu, Stair step, Jump rope.

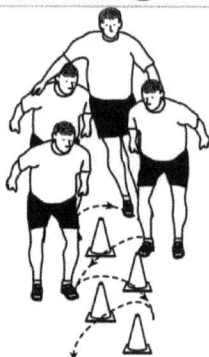

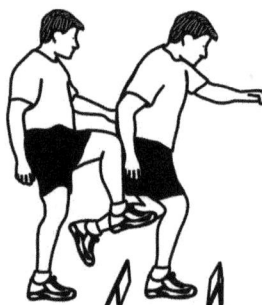

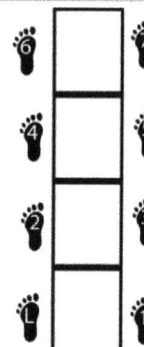

Balance Equipment

Can include **Foam rollers** *(also see Myofascial below)*

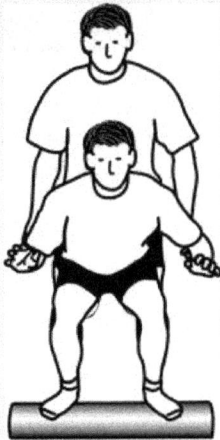

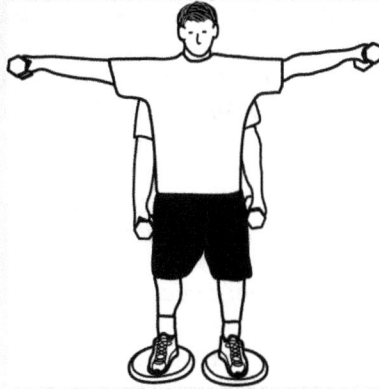

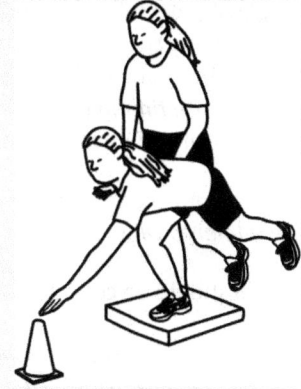

**Balance discs
Balance pad
Cones
Stepper
Bosu**

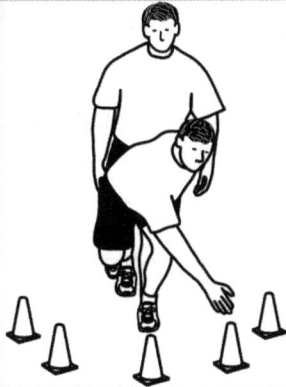

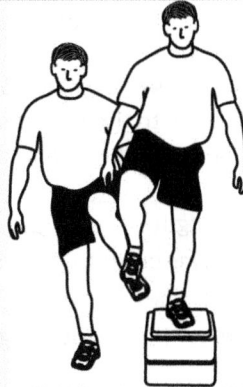

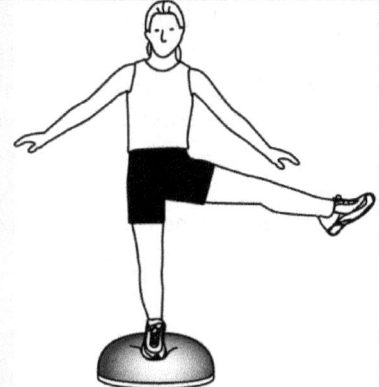

Exercise Bench (Optional)

The type really depends on what you will use it for. You can get a plain bench just for support (as above you can use a stability ball) or you can get all the bells and whistles. Some have pieces for leg extensions and curls, as well as arm pieces for butterflies. If you do not already have one, I suggest waiting until you start your exercise program and see what you feel you will need to advance.

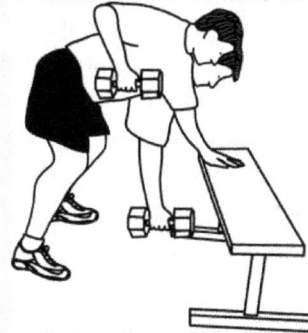

Examples For Myofascial

Massage Ball

Foam/Textured Rollers *(also see balance)*

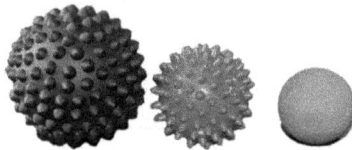

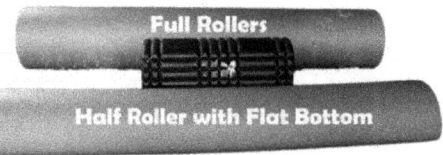

Full Rollers

Half Roller with Flat Bottom

Not Shown

- Exercise mat for floor exercises
- Ankle Weights
- Bed, couch or high table/mat
- Chair with/without arms - High or Low
- 10-inch play ball
- Pillow
- Towel roll
- Strap for stretches

SELF TESTS

Before starting the exercise program, it is a good idea to see where your baseline is. Taking the following tests will help guide you in the level you will need to start, and help progress by retaking the test periodically. *It is suggested to get a partner to help with both timing and safety, especially with balance tests.* The first 6 tests are modified versions starting at age 60 but are great for adults of any age. Tests 7-10 will help determine how quickly you can advance your balance program.

As with the exercises in this book, these tests should also be performed by those that are otherwise healthy with no chronic or acute ailments OR with supervision of a qualified health coach/personal trainer/physical therapist.

Tests 1-6 should be conducted in the following order if you are doing them at the same time.

A general warm up should be done prior to tests (*see Warm up/Cool down*).
- Stop immediately if any adverse reactions, such as nausea, dizziness, blurred vision, pain of any kind, chest pain, confusion or loss of muscle control.
- Stay hydrated, and do not proceed with testing on days with high temperature/humidity or any other conditions where you would not normally exercise.
- Practice each test several times before attempting to get an accurate score.
- It is advised that you have a second person to time the tests and make sure you are following proper form. Make sure your partner also understands the precautions and goals of these tests.

1. 30 second chair stand - Lower body strength
    o Needed for stair climbing, walking getting up out of tub/chair/car and reduce the risk of falls
2. 30 second arm curl test – Upper body strength
    o Needed to lift and carry everyday items, such as groceries and toolbox
3. 2-minute step test – Aerobic endurance
    o Needed for activities that require endurance, such as walking distance, grocery shopping and climbing stairs
4. Chair sit and reach – Lower body flexibility
    o Needed for normal gait patterns, correct posture, getting in/out of car/tub
5. Back stretch test – Shoulder flexibility
    o Needed to do various activities, such as combing hair and putting on overhead garments
6. 8 foot get up and go – Agility and dynamic balance
    o Needed for pretty much anything you do that requires getting up and walking, such as go to kitchen, bathroom or answering phone.
7. Narrow stance – Balance progression
8. Staggered stance – Balance progression
9. Tandem stance – Balance progression
10. One leg standing – Balance progression

TEST AND PURPOSE	PICTURE	EQUIPMENT NEEDED	EXPLANATION	RESULTS
30 Second Chair Stand Assess lower body strength *May not want to perform if any chronic pain or back issues. *If you are tall and have had a recent hip replacement skip this or use taller chair.		Straight back or folding chair (~17 inch height) against wall. Stopwatch, wrist watch or clock within view with second hand	*Sit with feet flat on the floor and arms crossed over the chest. *Get up to a full stand and then sit back down. ** Start the time – Immediately repeat as many *full stands* as you can in 30 seconds. *If you cannot stand with hands over chest, try pushing off on your thighs or get a chair with arms and push off arms. If using assist, make sure you note this for progression.*	**Normal Range repetitions** See table below

Normal Range repetitions

Age	Men	Women
60-64	14-19	12-17
65-69	12-18	11-16
70-74	12-17	10-15
75-79	11-17	10-15
80-84	10-15	9-14
85-89	8-14	8-13
90-94	7-12	4-11

TEST AND PURPOSE	PICTURE	EQUIPMENT NEEDED	EXPLANATION	RESULTS
30 Second Arm Curl Test Upper body strength		Straight back or folding chair without arms. Can be done in standing. Stopwatch or clock within view with second hand Women: 5 lb dumbbell Men: 8 lb dumbbell Can use a wrist weight if arthritis and cannot hold a dumbbell	*Sit with feet flat on the floor towards the edge seat towards dominant side. **Start with the arm extended by your side holding dumbbell in the dominant hand. *Bend elbow with palm facing you keeping the upper arm next to the body (elbow pressed into your side). *Return to starting position. *Keep the wrist straight – do not flex or extend the wrist. **Start the time – Immediately repeat as many arm curls as you can in 30 seconds *with proper form.* *If you cannot hold the suggested weight with proper form, use a lighter weight. Make sure you note this for progression.*	**Normal Range repetitions** See table below

Normal Range repetitions

Age	Men	Women
60-64	16-22	13-19
65-69	15-21	12-18
70-74	14-21	12-17
75-79	13-19	11-17
80-84	13-19	10-16
85-89	11-17	10-15
90-94	10-14	8-13

TEST AND PURPOSE	PICTURE	EQUIPMENT NEEDED	EXPLANATION	RESULTS
2 Minute Step Test Aerobic endurance		Wall for support and to mark step height. Sturdy chair to hold on opposite side if unsteady. Stopwatch or clock within view with second hand	*For accuracy, may need a second person to judge step height and count. *Step with side next to wall. Bring knee up mid-thigh between the knee and the hip. Mark the wall with tape at this height. This will be your minimum step height. *Practice marching in place to this step height. **Start the time – Immediately start marching (not jogging) for 2 minutes. Count the number of *full steps* (both legs) that come up to step height. Every time the right knee reaches proper step height; this is counted as one step. *If shortness of breath, extreme fatigue or unable to continue to step height, stop test and this is your baseline.* * *If unable to get to step height, but able to complete 2 minutes. Make sure you note this for progression.* *If unsteady, hold onto chair on opposite side for support.*	**Normal Range steps** <table><tr><td>Age</td><td>Men</td><td>Women</td></tr><tr><td>60-64</td><td>87-115</td><td>75-107</td></tr><tr><td>65-69</td><td>86-116</td><td>73-107</td></tr><tr><td>70-74</td><td>80-110</td><td>68-101</td></tr><tr><td>75-79</td><td>73-109</td><td>68-100</td></tr><tr><td>80-84</td><td>71-103</td><td>60-90</td></tr><tr><td>85-89</td><td>59-91</td><td>55-85</td></tr><tr><td>90-94</td><td>52-86</td><td>44-72</td></tr></table>

TEST AND PURPOSE	PICTURE	EQUIPMENT NEEDED	EXPLANATION	RESULTS
Chair Sit And Reach Lower body flexibility, *primarily hamstrings* *Do not do if recent hip replacement or severe osteoporosis. *Stretch to discomfort, not pain.		Chair (~17 inch height). Make sure chair is secure and does not tip forward. 18 inch ruler or yardstick	*Sit on the edge chair – you should feel the middle of the thigh at the edge of the chair. *Bend one leg with foot flat on floor. *Straighten the target leg in front with heel on the floor and foot flexed up. *Reach forward with one hand over the other and middle fingers even. *Exhale as you bend forward at the hips and reach forward towards or past the toes. Keep the extended knee straight and adjust if it bends. *Practice a few times on both legs to see which one you would prefer for testing. Do two tests and measure as below. **Measure tips of middle fingers to the tip of the shoe (closest to ½ inch). ***The midpoint at the toe of the shoe is considered zero (0), and is scored as such if you reach this point. ***If the reach is short, score this as a minus (-) ***If the reach is past this point, score this as a plus (+)	**Normal Range inches** See table below

Chair Sit And Reach — Normal Range inches

Age	Men	Women
60-64	-2.5 +4.0	-0.5 + 5.0
65-69	-3.0 +3.0	-0.5 + 4.5
70-74	-3.0 +3.0	-1.0 + 4.0
75-79	-4.0 +2.0	-1.5 + 3.5
80-84	-5.5 +1.5	2.0 + 3.0
85-89	-5.5 +0.5	-2.5 + 2.5
90-94	-6.5 -0.5	-4.5 + 1.0

TEST AND PURPOSE	PICTURE	EQUIPMENT NEEDED	EXPLANATION	RESULTS
Back Stretch Test Shoulder flexibility *Do not do if any upper back, shoulder or neck injuries		18-inch ruler or yardstick	*Will need second person to measure. *Stand and place the target arm over the same shoulder, palm down with fingers extended. Reach down the middle of the back. *Place the opposite arm around the back, palm up reaching up the middle of the back towards other hand. Try to touch middle fingers together or overlap if possible. *Do not overlap fingers and pull.* *Practice a few times on both arms to see which one you would prefer for testing. Do two tests and measure as below. **Measure the distance between tips of middle fingers or overlap. ***If the middle fingers do not touch, score this as a minus (-) ***If the middle fingers just touch, score this as a zero (0) ***If the middle fingers overlap, score this as a plus (+)	**Normal Range inches** See table below

Back Stretch Test — Normal Range inches

Age	Men	Women
60-64	-6.5 +0.0	-3.0 + 1.5
65-69	-7.5 -1.0	-3.5 + 1.5
70-74	-8.0 -1.0	-4.0 + 1.0
75-79	-9.0 -2.0	-5.0 + 0.5
80-84	-9.5 -2.0	-5.5 + 0.0
85-89	-9.5 -3.0	-7.0 -1.0
90-94	-10.5 -4.0	-8.0 -1.0

Self Tests

TEST AND PURPOSE	PICTURE	EQUIPMENT NEEDED	EXPLANATION	RESULTS		
8 Foot Get Up And Go Agility and dynamic balance *If unsteady, have someone by your side in case you lose your balance. 8 feet →		Chair against wall (~17-inch height) Cone or another marker to walk around Stopwatch or clock within view with second hand *Put chair against wall and cone 8 feet in front. Measure from front of chair to back of cone (side facing chair).	*This is done better with a partner watching the clock or a stopwatch. *Sit on chair, back straight, feet flat on floor, one foot slightly in front, torso leaning slightly forward and hands resting on thighs. **Start the time – Immediately get up and walk around the cone (either side) and return to chair. Stopwatch immediately when seated. **Try 2-3x and record the fastest time within 10th /second. *Can use a cane or walker or start from standing position. Make sure you note this for progression.	**Normal Range seconds**		
				Age	Men	Women
				60-64	5.6-3.8	6.0-4.4
				65-69	5.9-4.3	6.4-4.8
				70-74	6.2-4.4	7.1-4.9
				75-79	7.2-4.6	7.4-5.2
				80-84	7.6-5.2	8.7-5.7
				85-89	8.9-5.5	9.6-6.2
				90-94	10.0-6.2	11.5-7.3

TEST AND PURPOSE	PICTURE	EQUIPMENT NEEDED	EXPLANATION	RESULTS
Narrow Stance Balance progression		Wall, counter or chair within arm's reach for support if needed Stopwatch or clock within view with second hand	Keep your feet together and stand for up to one minute. *Time stops if loss of balance with need to hold on to support.	One minute: Normal *Progress to Staggered Stance Test* *Less than 30 seconds: Continue balance program with wider stance and progress to narrow stance using support. *(See Balance)*
Staggered Stance Balance progression		Wall, counter or chair within arm's reach for support if needed Stopwatch or clock within view with second hand	Stand with one foot in front of the other and slightly off to the side. Stand for up to one minute. Repeat on other side for comparison *Time stops if loss of balance with need to hold on to support.	One minute: Normal *Progress to Tandem Stance Test* *Less than 30 seconds: Continue balance program using support. *(See Balance)*
Tandem Stance Balance progression		Wall, counter or chair within arm's reach for support if needed Stopwatch or clock within view with second hand	Stand with one foot directly in back of the other – toe should be touching the opposite heel. Hold for up to one minute. Repeat on other side for comparison *Time stops if loss of balance with need to hold on to support.	One minute: Normal *Progress to One Leg Standing Balance* *Less than 30 seconds: Continue balance program using support. *(See Balance)*
Single Leg Stance Balance progression		Wall, counter or chair within arm's reach for support if needed Stopwatch or clock within view with second hand	Stand on one leg for up to one minute. Repeat on other side for comparison *Time stops if loss of balance with need to hold on to support or if opposite foot taps the floor	One minute: Normal *Less than 30 seconds: Continue balance program using support. *(See Balance)*

EXERCISE Myofascial Release	EXERCISE NUMBER	PAGE	REPS	SETS	X DAY	HOLD
ANTERIOR CHEST - BALL	1					
ANTERIOR CHEST - FOAM ROLL	2					
LATISSIMUS DORSI – BALL	3					
LATISSIMUS DORSI - FOAM ROLL	4					
TRICEP – FOAM ROLL	5					
OCCIPITAL RELEASE - FOAM ROLL	6					
THORACIC MOBILIZATION – SUPINE - FOAM ROLL	7					
THORACIC MOBILIZATION – STANDING - FOAM ROLL	8					
LUMBAR – STANDING – BALL - can do with foam roll	9					
LUMBAR – SUPINE – FOAM ROLLER	10					
HIP FLEXORS - BALL	11					
HIP FLEXORS – FOAM ROLL	12					
QUADRICEPS – BILATERAL - FOAM ROLL	13					
QUADRICEP – SINGLE - FOAM ROLL	14					
GLUTE /PIRIFORMIS - FOAM ROLL	15					
HIP ADDUCTORS – FOAM ROLL	16					
HAMSTRING – BILATERAL - FOAM ROLL	17					
HAMSTRING – SINGLE – FOAM ROLL	18					
CALVES – BILATERAL - FOAM ROLL	19					
CALVES – SINGLE - FOAM ROLL	20					
ILIOTIBIAL BAND (IT Band) - FOAM ROLL	21					
ILIOTIBIAL BAND (IT Band) - BALL	22					
PLANTAR FASCIA ROLLING – BALL	23					
PLANTAR FASCIA ROLLING - COLD SODA CAN	24					

EXERCISE Flexibility (Stretching)	EXERCISE NUMBER	PAGE	REPS	SETS	X DAY	HOLD
INVERSION	1					
EVERSION	2					
ANTERIOR TIBIALIS	3					
PLANTARFLEXION	4					
DORSIFLEXION - STRAP	5					
DORSIFLEXION - FLOOR ASSISTED	6					
STANDING CALF STRETCH - GASTROC	7					
STANDING CALF STRETCH - GASTROC – HAND ON KNEE	8					
GASTROCNEMIUS STAIR STRETCH	9					
STANDING CALF STRETCH - SOLEUS	10					
HAMSTRING STRETCH – TOWEL, BAND, STRAP or BELT	11					
HAMSTRING STRETCH – TOWEL, BAND, STRAP or BELT	12					
HAMSTRING STRETCH - TABLE, BED OR COUCH	13					
HAMSTRING / KNEE EXTENSION STRETCH - SEATED	14					
HAMSTRING STRETCH - STANDING	15					
TOE TOUCH – STANDING - NARROW or WIDE BOS	16					
HEEL SLIDES - SELF ASSISTED	17					
HEEL SLIDES - LONG SIT ASSISTED - TOWEL, BAND, STRAP or BELT	18					
HEEL SLIDES - SUPINE	19					
KNEE BENDS - EXERCISE BALL	20					
KNEE FLEXION – SELF ASSISTED - PRONE	21					
KNEE FLEXION – BELT ASSISTED - PRONE	22					
HEEL SLIDES - SELF ASSISTED	23					
HEEL SLIDES - SEATED	24					
KNEE FLEXION – SCOOT FORWARD - SEATED	25					

EXERCISE Flexibility (Stretching)	EXERCISE NUMBER	PAGE	REPS	SETS	X DAY	HOLD
KNEE FLEXION – STAIR OR STEP	26					
PIRIFORMIS STRETCH	27					
PIRIFORMIS STRETCH - EXERCISE BALL	28					
PIRIFORMIS STRETCH - LONG SIT	29					
PIRIFORMIS STRETCH – STANDING	30					
HIP FLEXOR STRETCH - SIDE OF BALL or CHAIR	31					
HIP FLEXOR STRETCH - STANDING	32					
HIP FLEXOR STRETCH - HALF KNEEL	33					
RUNNER'S STRETCH - MODIFIED	34					
HIP FLEXOR STRETCH – SUPINE	35					
HIP FLEXOR STRETCH – SUPINE - 2	36					
QUAD STRETCH - SIDELYING	37					
QUAD STRETCH - STANDING	38					
KNEE FALL OUT STRETCH or FROG STRETCH	39					
BUTTERFLY STRETCH	40					
HIP ADDUCTOR STRECH – KNEELING	41					
HIP ADDUCTOR STRECH - STANDING	42					
HIP EXTERNAL ROTATION STRETCH - SUPINE	43					
HIP INTERNAL ROTATION STRETCH - SEATED	44					
IT BAND STRETCH - STANDING	45					
IT BAND STRETCH -- SIDELYING	46					
NECK ROTATION and SIDE BENDS	47					
NECK FLEXION AND EXTENSION	48					
TRUNK FLEXION - SEATED	49					
LOW BACK STRETCH - SEATED	50					
LOW BACK STRETCH – STANDING - STRAIGHT & LATERAL	51					
LOW BACK STRETCH – RAIL OR DOORKNOB	52					

EXERCISE Flexibility (Stretching)	EXERCISE NUMBER	PAGE	REPS	SETS	X DAY	HOLD
PRAYER STRETCH and LATERAL	53					
PRAYER STRETCH - EXERCISE BALL	54					
CAT AND CAMEL	55					
KNEE TO CHEST STRETCH - SINGLE and BILATERAL	56					
PRONE ON ELBOWS	57					
PRESS UPS	58					
TRUNK ROTATION STRETCH – SINGLE LEG	59					
LOWER TRUNK ROTATIONS – BILATERAL	60					
TRUNK ROTATION - SEATED	61					
TRUNK ROTATION - STANDING or SEATED – DOWEL	62					
LATERAL TRUNK STRETCH - SINGLE, SEATED or STANDING	63					
LATERAL TRUNK STRETCH - BILATERAL SEATED or STANDING	64					
FLEXION - SUPINE - DOWEL	65					
WALL WALK	66					
FLEXION - TABLE SLIDE	67					
FLEXION - TABLE SLIDE - BALL	68					
EXTERNAL ROTATION - SUPINE – DOWEL *INTERNAL ROTATION ON OPPOSITE ARM*	69					
EXTERNAL ROTATION - 90-90 - DOWEL	70					
EXTERNAL ROTATION – SEATED – DOWEL *INTERNAL ROTATION ON OPPOSITE ARM*	71					
EXTERNAL ROTATION – STANDING – DOWEL *INTERNAL ROTATION ON OPPOSITE ARM*	72					
ABDUCTION - TABLE SLIDE - BALL	75					
ABDUCTION WITH DOWEL	76					
LYING DOWN EXTENSION - TABLE or BED	77					
WAND EXTENSION - STANDING	78					
CHEST STRETCH – SEATED, STANDING, or SUPINE	79					

EXERCISE **Flexibility (Stretching)**	EXERCISE NUMBER	PAGE	REPS	SETS	X DAY	HOLD
TRICEP STRETCH - STRAP or TOWEL	82					
POSTERIOR SHOULDER/DELTOID RELEASE	83					
POSTERIOR CAPSULE STRETCH	84					

Worksheets

EXERCISE Core / Stability	EXERCISE NUMBER	PAGE	REPS	SETS	X DAY	HOLD
ABDOMINAL BRACING TRAINING	1					
ABDOMINAL BRACING - SUPINE	2					
PELVIC TILT - SUPINE	3					
PELVIC TILT - KNEELING	4					
BRIDGING	5					
BRIDGE - BOSU	6					
BRIDGING WITH PILLOW SQUEEZE	7					
BRIDGING WITH PILLOW SQUEEZE - BOSU	8					
BRACE SUPINE MARCHING / BRIDGE LEG UP	9					
BRIDGE LEG UP - BOSU -	10					
SINGLE LEG BRIDGE	11					
BRIDGE SINGLE LEG - BOSU	12					
BRIDGING CROSSED LEG	13					
BRIDGING CROSSED LEG – BOSU	14					
BRIDGING CROSSED LEG - ARMS UP	15					
BRIDGING CROSSED LEG - ARMS UP - BOSU	16					
BRIDGE - ELASTIC BAND	17					
BRIDGING - ABDUCTION - ELASTIC BAND	18					
FLOOR BRIDGE - EXERCISE BALL	19					
FLOOR BRIDGE ALTERNATE LEG LIFT - EXERCISE BALL	20					
BRIDGE UPPER BACK - EXERCISE BALL	21					
BRIDGE UPPER BACK - SINGLE LEG - EXERCISE BALL	22					
QUADRUPED ALTERNATE ARM	23					
QUADRUPED ALTERNATE LEG	24					
QUADRUPED ALTERNATE ARM AND LEG	25					
BIRD DOG ELBOW TOUCHES	26					

EXERCISE	EXERCISE NUMBER	PAGE	REPS	SETS	X DAY	HOLD
Core / Stability						
PRONE BALL	27					
PRONE BALL - ALTERNATE ARM	28					
PRONE BALL - ALTERNATE LEG	29					
PRONE BALL - ALTERNATE ARM AND LEG	30					
MODIFIED PLANK	31					
MODIFIED PLANK - ALTERNATE LEG	32					
FULL PLANK	33					
PLANK - ALTERNATE ARMS	34					
PLANK - ALTERNATE LEGS	35					
PLANK - EXERCISE BALL	36					
PRONE ON ELBOWS	37					
PRESS UPS	38					
SKYDIVER	39					
PRONE SUPERMAN - BOSU	40					
TRUNK EXTENSION - BOSU	41					
TRUNK EXTENSION - HANDS CROSSED IN FRONT - BOSU	43					
SUPERMAN - ARMS BACK- EXERCISE BALL	44					
SUPERMAN – BOTH ARMS IN FRONT - EXERCISE BALL	45					
SUPERMAN – ONE ARM FORWARD / ONE ARM BACK - EXERCISE BALL	46					
LATERAL PLANK MODIFIED	47					
LATERAL PLANK MODIFIED- BOSU	48					
LATERAL PLANK - 1 KNEE 1 FOOT	49					
LATERAL PLANK - 1 KNEE 1 FOOT – BOSU	50					
LATERAL PLANK	51					
LATERAL PLANK - BOSU	52					

Worksheets

EXERCISE Core / Stability	EXERCISE NUMBER	PAGE	REPS	SETS	X DAY	HOLD
LEAN BACK	53					
LEAN BACK - BOSU	54					
LEAN BACK WITH ARMS OUT	55					
LEAN BACK WITH ARMS OUT - BOSU	56					
LEAN BACK WITH TWIST	57					
LEAN BACK WITH TWIST – BOSU	58					
CRUNCHY FROG	59					
SEATED BIKE - FORWARD AND BACKWARDS	60					
CRUNCH – ARMS OUT	61					
CRUNCH – ARMS OUT - BOSU	62					
CRUNCH – ARMS IN BACK OF HEAD	63					
CRUNCH – ARMS IN BACK OF HEAD - BOSU	64					
OBLIQUE CRUNCH	65					
OBLIQUE CRUNCH - BOSU	66					
90 DEGREE CRUNCH	67					
BALL CRUNCH – Can put legs on seat of chair	68					
CURL UPS – ARMS ON LEGS - EXERCISE BALL	69					
CURL UPS- ARMS CROSSED IN FRONT - EXERCISE BALL	70					
CURL UPS – ARMS BEHIND HEAD - EXERCISE BALL	71					
SUPINE CRUNCH TOUCH - EXERCISE BALL	72					
LOWER ABDOMINAL CRUNCH – WITH or WITHOUT BALL	73					
HIGH MARCH CRUNCH	74					
STANDING SIDE CRUNCH	75					
STANDING BIKE CRUNCH	76					

EXERCISE Lower Extremity - Lying & Seated Strengthening and Range of Motion	EXERCISE NUMBER	PAGE	REPS	SETS	X DAY	HOLD
INVERSION – SEATED - ELASTIC BAND	1					
INVERSION – SEATED - ELASTIC BAND - 2	2					
EVERSION – SEATED - ELASTIC BAND	3					
EVERSION – SEATED - ELASTIC BAND - 2	4					
ANKLE PUMPS - SEATED	5					
ANKLE PUMPS – SUPINE or FEET UP ON STOOL	6					
DORSIFLEXION – SEATED - ELASTIC BAND	7					
DORSIFLEXION – SEATED - ELASTIC BAND - 2	8					
PLANTARFLEXION - STRAP	9					
PLANTARFLEXION - SEATED – ELASTIC BAND	10					
HEEL SLIDES - SUPINE	11					
HEEL SLIDES - RESISTED EXTENSION – ELASTIC BAND	12					
QUAD SET –ISOMETRIC	13					
QUAD SET WITH TOWEL UNDER HEEL - ISOMETRIC	14					
SHORT ARC QUAD (SAQ) – SELF ASSISTED	15					
SHORT ARC QUAD - (SAQ)	16					
KNEE EXTENSION - SELF ASSISTED	17					
PARTIAL ARC QUAD - LOW SEAT	18					
LONG ARC QUAD (LAQ) – LOW SEAT (90 deg)	19					
LONG ARC QUAD (LAQ) – LOW SEAT - ANKLE WEIGHTS	20					
LONG ARC QUAD (LAQ) - HIGH SEAT	21					
LONG ARC QUAD (LAQ) - HIGH SEAT - ANKLE WEIGHTS	22					
LONG ARC QUAD - ELASTIC BAND – HAND HELD	23					
LONG ARC QUAD - ELASTIC BAND	24					

EXERCISE Lower Extremity - Lying & Seated Strengthening and Range of Motion	EXERCISE NUMBER	PAGE	REPS	SETS	X DAY	HOLD
HAMSTRING CURLS - PRONE - ASSISTED	25					
HAMSTRING CURLS - PRONE	26					
HAMSTRING CURLS - - PRONE - WEIGHTS	27					
HAMSTRING CURLS – PRONE - ELASTIC BAND	28					
HAMSTRING CURLS – ELASTIC BAND	29					
HAMSTRING CURLS – ELASTIC BAND - 2	30					
HAMSTRING CURLS ON BALL	31					
HAMSTRING CURLS - SINGLE LEG - EXERCISE BALL	32					
HIP FLEXION ISOMETRIC	33					
HIP FLEXION ISOMETRIC BILATERAL	34					
HIP FLEXION – ISOMETRIC	35					
STRAIGHT LEG RAISE (SLR)	36					
STRAIGHT LEG RAISE (SLR) – ANKLE WEIGHTS	37					
STRAIGHT LEG RAISE (SLR) - ELASTIC BAND	38					
SEATED MARCHING	39					
SEATED MARCHING - ELASTIC BAND	40					
HIP EXTENSION - PRONE	41					
HIP EXTENSION – PRONE – ANKLE WEIGHTS	42					
HIP EXTENSION – PRONE – ELASTIC BAND	43					
HIP EXTENSION – QUADRUPED	44					
HIP ABDUCTION - SUPINE	45					
HIP ABDUCTION - SUPINE – ANKLE WEIGHTS	46					
HIP ABDUCTION – SUPINE - ELASTIC BAND	47					
HIP ABDUCTION / CLAMS– SUPINE - ELASTIC BAND	48					
MODIFIED HIP ABDUCTION – SIDELYING	49					

EXERCISE Lower Extremity - Lying & Seated Strengthening and Range of Motion	EXERCISE NUMBER	PAGE	REPS	SETS	X DAY	HOLD
HIP ABDUCTION – SIDELYING	50					
HIP ABDUCTION – SIDELYING - WEIGHTS	51					
HIP ABDUCTION – SIDELYING - ELASTIC BAND	52					
CLAM SHELLS	53					
SIDELYING CLAM - ELASTIC BAND	54					
HIP ABDUCTION - FIRE HYDRANT - QUADRUPED	55					
HIP ABDUCTION - FIRE HYDRANT – QUADRUPED - ELASTIC BAND	56					
HIP ABDUCTION - SEATED - STRAIGHT LEG	57					
HIP ABDUCTION - SEATED - STRAIGHT LEG – ANKLE WEIGHT	58					
HIP ABDUCTION - SINGLE- SEATED	59					
HIP ABDUCTION - SINGLE- SEATED – ELASTIC BAND	60					
HIP ABDUCTION - BILATERAL- SEATED	61					
HIP ABDUCTION - BILATERAL- SEATED - ELASTIC BAND	62					
HIP ADDUCTION SQUEEZE – SUPINE – KNEES BENT	63					
HIP ADDUCTION SQUEEZE – SUPINE – LEGS STRAIGHT	64					
HIP ADDUCTION - SIDELYING	65					
INTERNAL ROTATION - HEEL SQUEEZE - ISOMETRIC	67					
HIP INTERNAL ROTATION - SUPINE	68					
REVERSE CLAMS - SIDELYING	69					
REVERSE CLAMS - SIDELYING - ELASTIC BAND	70					
HIP INTERNAL ROTATION - SEATED	71					
HIP INTERNAL ROTATION - ELASTIC BAND	72					
HIP EXTERNAL ROTATION - SUPINE	73					

Worksheets

EXERCISE Lower Extremity - Lying & Seated Strengthening and Range of Motion	EXERCISE NUMBER	PAGE	REPS	SETS	X DAY	HOLD
HIP EXTERNAL ROTATION - ELASTIC BAND	74					
HIP ROTATIONS – BILATERAL - SIDELYING	75					
HIP ROTATION - SEATED - BALL and ELASTIC BAND	76					
PRESS – BILATERAL – ELASTIC BAND	77					
PRESS – SINGLE LEG – ELASTIC BAND	78					
HIP HIKE - STANDING	79					
HIP HIKE – KNEELING	80					
GLUTE SETS - PRONE	81					
GLUTE SET - SUPINE	82					
GLUTE SQUEEZE - SITTING	83					
GLUTE SCULPT (MAX/MEDIUS)	84					

Worksheets

EXERCISE Upper Extremity Strengthening and Range of Motion	EXERCISE NUMBER	PAGE	REPS	SETS	X DAY	HOLD
ELBOW FLEXION EXTENSION - SUPINE	1					
ELBOW FLEXION / EXTENSION - GRAVITY ELIMINATED	2					
BICEPS CURLS – ALTERNATING	3					
BICEPS CURL - SELF FIXATION – ELASTIC BAND	4					
SEATED BICEPS CURLS - ALTERNATING	5					
SEATED BICEPS CURLS - BILATERAL	6					
CONCENTRATION CURLS – SITTING	7					
PREACHER CURL ON BALL	8					
BICEPS CURLS	9					
BICEPS CURLS - RADIOBRACHIALIS - HAMMER CURL	10					
BICEPS CURLS - BRACHIALIS	11					
BICEPS CURLS – ROTATE OUTWARD	12					
BICEPS CURLS – ONE ARM - ELASTIC BAND	13					
BICEPS CURLS – BILATERAL - ELASTIC BAND	14					
BICEPS CURLS - RADIOBRACHIALIS - HAMMER CURL – ONE ARM - ELASTIC BAND	15					
BICEPS CURLS - RADIOBRACHIALIS - HAMMER CURL – BILATERAL - ELASTIC BAND	16					
BICEPS CURLS – BRACHIALIS - ONE ARM - ELASTIC BAND	17					
BICEPS CURL – BRACHIALIS – BILATERAL - ELASTIC BAND	18					
TRICEPS - SELF FIXATION - ELASTIC BAND	19					
OVERHEAD TRICEPS - SELF FIXATION –SEATED OR STANDING - ELASTIC BAND	20					
TRICEP EXTENSION – SITTING OR STANDING - WEIGHT	21					
TRICEP EXTENSION – SITTING OR STANDING – BILATERAL - WEIGHT	22					
ELBOW EXTENSION - BALL	23					

EXERCISE **Upper Extremity** **Strengthening and Range of Motion**	EXERCISE NUMBER	PAGE	REPS	SETS	X DAY	HOLD
ELBOW EXTENSION - SKULL CRUSHER - BALL	24					
TRICEPS - ELASTIC BAND	25					
TRICEPS - BENT OVER	26					
CHAIR DIPS / PUSH UPS	27					
DIPS OFF CHAIR	28					
PENDULUM SHOULDER FORWARD/BACK	29					
PENDULUM SHOULDER – SIDE TO SIDE	30					
PENDULUM SHOULDER CIRCLES	31					
PENDULUMS - SUPINE	32					
ISOMETRIC FLEXION	33					
SHOULDER FLEXION – SIDELYING	34					
FLEXION – SUPINE - SINGLE OR BILATERAL	35					
FLEXION – SUPINE – SINGLE OR BILATERAL - WEIGHT	36					
FLEXION – SUPINE - DOWEL	37					
FLEXION – SUPINE - DOWEL - Weight	38					
FLEXION - SELF FIXATION – ELASTIC BAND	39					
FLEXION – ELASTIC BAND	40					
FLEXION - STANDING - PALMS DOWN / OVERHAND DOWEL	41					
FLEXION - STANDING - PALMS UP / UNDERHAND DOWEL	42					
FLEXION – PALMS FACING INWARD	43					
FLEXION – PALMS DOWN	44					
V RAISE	45					
V RAISE – WEIGHTS	46					
MILITARY PRESS – DOWEL	47					
MILITARY PRESS - FREE WEIGHTS	48					

EXERCISE Upper Extremity Strengthening and Range of Motion	EXERCISE NUMBER	PAGE	REPS	SETS	X DAY	HOLD
ISOMETRIC EXTENSION	49					
PRONE EXTENSION - EXERCISE BALL	50					
SHOULDER EXTENSION - STANDING	51					
SHOULDER EXTENSION - STANDING - WEIGHTS	52					
EXTENSION – STANDING – DOWEL	53					
EXTENSION - SELF FIXATION - ELASTIC BAND	54					
EXTENSION - ELASTIC BAND	55					
EXTENSION - BILATERAL - ELASTIC BAND	56					
INTERNAL ROTATION – ISOMETRIC	57					
INTERNAL ROTATION - ISOMETRIC- ELEVATED	58					
INTERNAL ROTATION - SIDELYING	59					
INTERNAL ROTATION - ELASTIC BAND	60					
INTERNAL / EXTERNAL ROTATION - STANDING – DOWEL	61					
INTERNAL ROTATION – DOWEL	62					
EXTERNAL ROTATION - ISOMETRIC	63					
EXTERNAL ROTATION - ISOMETRIC – ELEVATED	64					
EXTERNAL ROTATION WITH TOWEL - SIDELYING	65					
EXTERNAL ROTATION – 90/90 - WEIGHTS	66					
EXTERNAL ROTATION - BILATERAL - ELASTIC BAND	67					
EXTERNAL ROTATION - ELASTIC BAND	68					
ADDUCTION – ISOMETRIC	69					
ADDUCTION - ELASTIC BAND	70					
ABDUCTION – ISOMETRIC	71					
HORIZONTAL ABDUCTION - DOWEL	72					

Worksheets

EXERCISE Upper Extremity Strengthening and Range of Motion	EXERCISE NUMBER	PAGE	REPS	SETS	X DAY	HOLD
HORIZONTAL ABDUCTION/ADDUCTTION - SUPINE	73					
HORIZONTAL ABDUCTION/ADDUCTTION - SUPINE -WEIGHT	74					
ABDUCTION - SIDELYING	75					
HORIZONTAL ABDUCTION - SIDELYING	76					
ABDUCTION – WEIGHT	77					
ABDUCTION – ELASTIC BAND	78					
HORIZONTAL ABDUCTION – BILATERAL - ELASTIC BAND	79					
90/90 ABDUCTION - WEIGHT	80					
LATERAL RAISES	81					
LATERAL RAISES – LEAN FORWARD	82					
LATERAL RAISES – LEAN FORWARD - ARM ROTATION	83					
FRONTAL RAISE – WEIGHTS	84					
UPRIGHT ROW – WEIGHTS	85					
UPRIGHT ROW – ELASTIC BAND	86					
SHRUGS	87					
SHRUGS - WEIGHTS	88					
SHOULDER ROLLS	89					
SHOULDER ROLLS - WEIGHTS	90					
SCAPULAR RETRACTIONS - BILATERAL	91					
SCAPULAR RETRACTION – SINGLE ARM	92					
ELASTIC BAND SCAPULAR RETRACTIONS WITH MINI SHOULDER EXTENSIONS	93					
PRONE RETRACTION	94					
SCAPULAR PROTRACTION - SUPINE - BILATERAL	95					
SCAPULAR PROTRACTION - SUPINE - WEIGHT	96					

EXERCISE **Upper Extremity** **Strengthening and Range of Motion**	EXERCISE NUMBER	PAGE	REPS	SETS	X DAY	HOLD
SCAPULAR PROTRACTION - SUPINE - ELASTIC BAND	97					
SCAPULAR PROTRACTION / TABLE PLANK	98					
CHEST PRESS – SEATED or STANDING - ELASTIC BAND	99					
CHEST PRESS – BALL, FLOOR or BENCH- WEIGHTS	100					
DOWEL PRESS – STANDING	101					
CHEST PRESS – STANDING or SEATED	102					
BENT OVER ROWS	103					
ROWS – PRONE	104					
ROWS - ELASTIC BAND	105					
WIDE ROWS - ELASTIC BAND	106					
LOW ROW – ELASTIC BAND	107					
HIGH ROW – ELASTIC BAND	108					
FLY'S – FLOOR - WEIGHT	109					
FLY'S – BALL or BENCH – WEIGHT	110					
WALL PUSH UPS	111					
WALL PUSH UP - BALL	112					
WALL PUSH UP - Triceps uneven	113					
WALL PUSH UP - Hands inverted	114					
WALL PUSH UP - Narrow	115					
WALL PUSH UP – Wide	116					
PUSH UPS - BALL	117					
PUSH UP - MODIFIED	118					
PUSH UP	119					
PUSH UP -DIAMOND	120					
PUSH UP – MODIFIED - BOSU - UNSTABLE	121					

EXERCISE Upper Extremity Strengthening and Range of Motion	EXERCISE NUMBER	PAGE	REPS	SETS	X DAY	HOLD
PUSH UP – BOSU - UNSTABLE	122					
PUSH UP – MODIFIED – INVERTED BOSU - UNSTABLE	123					
PUSH UP – INVERTED BOSU - UNSTABLE	124					

EXERCISE Balance / Standing Exercises	EXERCISE NUMBER	PAGE	REPS	SETS	X DAY	HOLD
WIDE BOS DECREASING TO NARROW BOS	1					
NARROW BOS	2					
ARM MOVEMENT	3					
TRUNK ROTATION	4					
EYES SHUTS	5					
HEAD TURNS	6					
READING ALOUD	7					
BALANCE PAD	8					
SPLIT STANCE – SEMI TANDEM	9					
SPLIT STANCE - Progression	10					
TANDEM- SHARPENED ROMBERG STANCE	11					
TANDEM STANCE - Progression	12					
SINGLE LEG STANCE (SLS)	13					
SINGLE LEG STANCE (SLS) - Progression	14					
SLS – LEG FORWARD	15					
SLS – LEG BACKWARDS	16					
SLS – LEG FORWARD / OPPOSITE ARM UP	17					
SLS – LEG BACKWARDS / OPPOSITE ARM UP	18					
SLS - REACH FORWARD	19					
SLS - REACH TWIST	20					
SINGLE LEG TOE TAP	21					
SINGLE LEG STANCE - CLOCKS	22					
BALL ROLLS - HEEL TOE	23					
BALL ROLLS - LATERAL	24					
SQUAT	25					
SIT TO STAND	26					

Worksheets

EXERCISE Balance / Standing Exercises	EXERCISE NUMBER	PAGE	REPS	SETS	X DAY	HOLD
SQUATS – WALL WITH BALL	27					
SQUATS WITH WEIGHTS	28					
MINI SQUAT - UNSTABLE SUPPORT - FOAM PAD	29					
SQUATS - SINGLE LEG	30					
SIDE TO SIDE WEIGHT SHIFT	31					
FORWARD AND BACKWARDS WEIGHT SHIFTS	32					
SPLIT STANCE WEIGHT SHIFT SIDE TO SIDE	33					
SPLIT STANCE WEIGHT SHIFT FORWARD AND BACKWARDS	34					
WALL FALLS - FORWARD - BALANCE DRILL	35					
WALL FALLS - LATERAL - BALANCE DRILL	36					
WALL FALLS - BACKWARDS - BALANCE DRILL	37					
WALL FALLS - SINGLE LEG - FORWARD - BALANCE DRILL	38					
WALL FALLS - SINGLE LEG - LATERAL - BALANCE DRILL	39					
WALL FALLS - SINGLE LEG - MEDIAL - BALANCE DRILL	40					
WALL FALLS - SINGLE LEG - BACKWARDS - BALANCE DRILL	41					
FALL LATERAL - STEP RECOVERY	42					
FALL FORWARD - STEP RECOVERY	43					
FALL BACKWARD - STEP RECOVERY	44					
TOE TAP ABDUCTION	45					
HIP ABDUCTION - STANDING	46					
HIP EXTENSION – STANDING	47					
HIP FLEXION - STANDING – STRAIGHT LEG RAISE	48					
HIP / KNEE FLEXION - SINGLE LEG	49					
STANDING MARCHING	50					

EXERCISE Balance / Standing Exercises	EXERCISE NUMBER	PAGE	REPS	SETS	X DAY	HOLD
HAMSTRING CURL	51					
TOE RAISES	52					
TOE RAISES IR AND ER	53					
ONE LEGGED TOE RAISE	54					
SINGLE LEG BALANCE FORWARD	55					
SINGLE LEG BALANCE LATERAL	56					
SINGLE LEG BALANCE RETRO	57					
SINGLE LEG STANCE RETROLATERAL	58					
SQUAT	59					
SINGLE LEG SQUAT	60					
LUNGE – STATIC	61					
LUNGE FORWARD/BACKWARD	62					
FOUR CORNER MARCHING IN PLACE	63					
FOUR CORNER MARCHING IN PLACE WITH HEAD TURNS	64					
WALKING ON HEELS FORWARD AND BACKWARDS	65					
WALKING ON TOES FORWARD AND BACKWARDS	66					
TANDEM STANCE AND WALK – FORWARD AND BACKWARDS	67					
RUNNING MAN	68					
HOP STICK - FORWARD	69					
HOP STICK - BACKWARDS	70					
MINI LATERAL LUNGE	71					
SIDE STEPPING	72					
HOP STICK - LATERAL	73					
SINGLE LEG DEAD LIFT	74					

EXERCISE	EXERCISE NUMBER	PAGE	REPS	SETS	X DAY	HOLD
Balance / Standing Exercises						
CONE TAPS - SINGLE LEG STANCE	75					
CONE TAPS - SINGLE LEG STANCE - UNSTABLE	76					
FIGURE 8 AROUND CONES	77					
FIGURE 8 AROUND CONES – FOOT OR HAND TAP	78					
BALANCE DOUBLE LEG STANCE - WIDE	79					
BALANCE DOUBLE LEG STANCE - NARROW	80					
TANDEM STANCE	81					
TANDEM WALK	82					
SINGLE LEG STANCE - ABDUCTION	83					
SINGLE LEG STANCE - ABDUCTION	84					
SINGLE LEG STANCE – FORWARD KICK	85					
SINGLE LEG STANCE – HAMSTRING CURL	86					
SINGLE LEG SQUAT – LEG FORWARD	87					
SINGLE LEG SQUAT – LEG BACKWARDS	88					
TOE TAP OR HEEL PLACEMENT	89					
PULL UP FOOT TOUCHES ON STEP	90					
ALTERNATING SUSTAINED FOOT TOUCHES ON STEP	91					
STEP UP AND OVER	92					
FORWARD SWING THROUGH STEP	93					
SIDE STEPPING - *REPEAT STEPS 89-93 from a side approach.*	94					

Worksheets

EXERCISE Agility/Reactivity/Speed	EXERCISE NUMBER	PAGE	REPS	SETS	X DAY	HOLD
Four Square Drills	1					
Dots	2					
Ladder Drills	3					
Box Drills	4					
Cones	5					
Hurdles	6					

Myofascial Release

Myofascial release (MFR, self-myofascial release) is an alternative medicine therapy that claims to treat skeletal muscle immobility and pain by relaxing contracted muscles, improving blood and lymphatic circulation, and stimulating the stretch reflex in muscles.

Fascia is a thin, tough, elastic type of connective tissue that wraps most structures within the human body, including muscle. Fascia supports and protects these structures. Osteopathic theory proposes that this soft tissue can become restricted due to psychogenic disease, overuse, trauma, infectious agents, or inactivity, often resulting in pain, muscle tension, and corresponding diminished blood flow. (Wikipedia - *https://en.wikipedia.org/wiki/Myofascial_release*)

Possible Benefits of Myofascial Release

- Muscle relaxation
- Improves muscular and joint range of motion
- Reduces muscle soreness and improves tissue recovery
- Encourages the flow of lymph.
- Improves neuromuscular efficiency.
- Reduces adhesions and scar tissue.
- Releases trigger point (sensitivity and pain) – brings in blood flow and nutrient exchange.
- Maintains normal functional muscular length / Provides optimal length-tension relationship.
- Corrects muscle imbalances

USE

- Roll on foam roller or ball until you find the sore spot or trigger point. When you find this point, stop and rest on it or decrease the range to this particular area and hold for 10-20 seconds.
- Apply pressure to muscle area only. Try not to roll over bones, joints or directly on the spine (you can use a ball over the muscles on the side of the spine).
- Use this as a part of your warmup for particular areas you are exercising that day (for instance the hamstrings, calves and quadricep on leg strengthening day)
- You can use this technique on additional days for trouble areas and can even devote a dedicated session for whole body myofascial release.

Equipment Needed: FOAM ROLLER and/or TEXTURED or SOFT MASSAGE BALL

EXERCISE Myofascial Release	EXERCISE NUMBER	NOTES
ANTERIOR CHEST - BALL	1	
ANTERIOR CHEST - FOAM ROLL	2	
LATISSIMUS DORSI – BALL	3	
LATISSIMUS DORSI - FOAM ROLL	4	
TRICEP – FOAM ROLL	5	
OCCIPITAL RELEASE - FOAM ROLL	6	
THORACIC MOBILIZATION – SUPINE - FOAM ROLL	7	
THORACIC MOBILIZATION – STANDING - FOAM ROLL	8	
LUMBAR – STANDING – BALL - can do with foam roll	9	
LUMBAR – SUPINE – FOAM ROLLER	10	
HIP FLEXORS - BALL	11	
HIP FLEXORS – FOAM ROLL	12	
QUADRICEPS – BILATERAL - FOAM ROLL	13	
QUADRICEP – SINGLE - FOAM ROLL	14	
GLUTE /PIRIFORMIS - FOAM ROLL	15	
HIP ADDUCTORS – FOAM ROLL	16	
HAMSTRING – BILATERAL - FOAM ROLL	17	
HAMSTRING – SINGLE – FOAM ROLL	18	
CALVES – BILATERAL - FOAM ROLL	19	
CALVES – SINGLE - FOAM ROLL	20	
ILIOTIBIAL BAND (IT Band) - FOAM ROLL	21	
ILIOTIBIAL BAND (IT Band) - BALL	22	
PLANTAR FASCIA ROLLING – BALL	23	
PLANTAR FASCIA ROLLING - COLD SODA CAN	24	

Myofascial Release

	_____ Reps _____ Sets _____X Day _____Hold		_____ Reps _____ Sets _____X Day _____Hold
1	**Notes:**	**2**	**Notes:**

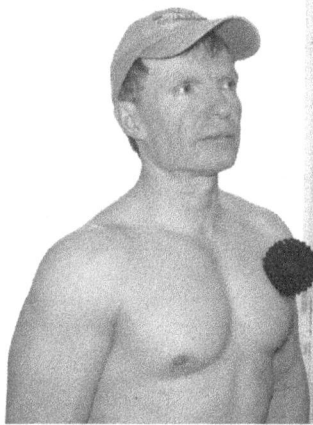

ANTERIOR CHEST - BALL

Face towards the wall and place small ball at the outside of chest. Bend knees up and down to find the target point and hold.

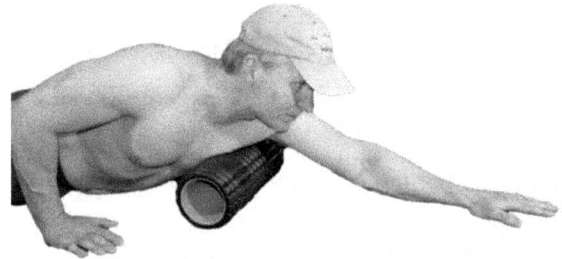

ANTERIOR CHEST - FOAM ROLL

Lie face down so that a foam roll is under the upper part of your arm and chest. Using your other arm and legs, roll forward and back across this area.

	_____ Reps _____ Sets _____X Day _____Hold		_____ Reps _____ Sets _____X Day _____Hold
3	**Notes:**	**4**	**Notes:**

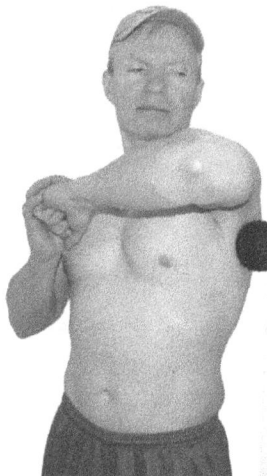

LATISSIMUS DORSI – BALL

Turn with your target side towards the wall and place small ball on the side under the shoulder. Bend knees up and down to find the target point and hold.

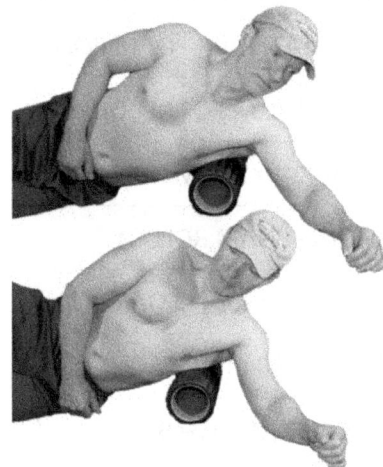

LATISSIMUS DORSI - FOAM ROLL

Lie on your side so that a foam roll is under the upper part of your arm and back. Using your other arm and legs, roll forward and back across this area.

	_____ Reps _____ Sets _____ X Day _____ Hold		_____ Reps _____ Sets _____ X Day _____ Hold
5	Notes:	**6**	Notes:

TRICEP – FOAM ROLL

In a sidelying position, place your tricep on the foam roll. Use the opposite arm and your body to help roll out the arm on the foam roll.

OCCIPITAL RELEASE - FOAM ROLL

Lie on your back and put a foam roll under the back of your head. Turn your head slowly from side to side.

	_____ Reps _____ Sets _____ X Day _____ Hold		_____ Reps _____ Sets _____ X Day _____ Hold
7	Notes:	**8**	Notes:

THORACIC MOBILIZATION – SUPINE - FOAM ROLL

Lie on a foam roller. While supporting your neck, roll up and down your mid-back.

THORACIC MOBILIZATION – STANDING - FOAM ROLL

Stand with a foam roll behind your upper back. Slowly perform mini-squats and allow the foam roller to roll up and down your back for a self-massage.

	_____ Reps _____ Sets _____ X Day _____ Hold
9	Notes:

LUMBAR – STANDING – BALL - can do with foam roll

Place small ball in lower back on the side of the spine. DO NOT roll directly over the spine. Slowly perform mini-squats and allow the ball to roll up and down your back for a self-massage.
*Can use foam roll behind lower back and follow above directions.

	_____ Reps _____ Sets _____ X Day _____ Hold
10	Notes:

LUMBAR – SUPINE – FOAM ROLLER

Lie on a foam roll under the lower back. While supporting your upper body, roll up and down your lower back.

	_____ Reps _____ Sets _____ X Day _____ Hold
11	Notes:

HIP FLEXORS - BALL   **Ball under hip flexor**

Lie on your stomach and place small ball under hip flexor. Roll up and down ball making small movements and hold on the target muscle.

	_____ Reps _____ Sets _____ X Day _____ Hold
12	Notes:

HIP FLEXORS – FOAM ROLL

Lie on your stomach and place foam roll under both hip flexors. Roll up and down avoiding rolling directly over hip bones.

13	_____ Reps _____ Sets _____ X Day _____ Hold	
	Notes:	

QUADRICEPS – BILATERAL - FOAM ROLL

Lie face down so that a foam roll is under the top of your thighs. Using your arms propped on your elbows, roll forward and back across this area.

14	_____ Reps _____ Sets _____ X Day _____ Hold	
	Notes:	

QUADRICEP – SINGLE - FOAM ROLL

Lie face down so that a foam roll is under the top of your target thigh. Cross your other leg over the top of your target leg. Using your arms propped on your elbows, roll forward and back across this area.

15	_____ Reps _____ Sets _____ X Day _____ Hold	
	Notes:	

GLUTE /PIRIFORMIS - FOAM ROLL

Sit on a foam roll and cross your affected leg on top of your other knee. Lean slightly towards your target side. Using your arms and unaffected leg roll forward and back across your buttock area.

16	_____ Reps _____ Sets _____ X Day _____ Hold	
	Notes:	

HIP ADDUCTORS – FOAM ROLL

Lie on your stomach supported by arms and lace your inner thigh on the roller. Roll and compress the target thigh muscle.

_____ Reps _____ Sets _____ X Day _____ Hold	_____ Reps _____ Sets _____ X Day _____ Hold
17 Notes:	**18** Notes:

HAMSTRING – BILATERAL - FOAM ROLL

Sit on a foam roll under both thighs. Using your arms, roll forward and back across this area

HAMSTRING – SINGLE – FOAM ROLL

Sit on a foam roll under thigh. Using your arms, roll forward and back across this area.

_____ Reps _____ Sets _____ X Day _____ Hold	_____ Reps _____ Sets _____ X Day _____ Hold
19 Notes:	**20** Notes:

CALVES – BILATERAL - FOAM ROLL

Sit with the foam roll under your both your calves. Lift your body up with your arms and roll forward and back across your calf area. Try turning toes in and out to access the inside and outside of calf areas. Do not roll in the crease of your knee.

CALVES – SINGLE - FOAM ROLL

Sit with the foam roll under your target calf and cross your other leg on top. Lift your body up with your arms and roll forward and back across your calf area. Do not roll in the crease of your knee.

	_____ Reps _____ Sets _____X Day _____Hold		_____ Reps _____ Sets _____X Day _____Hold
21	Notes:	**22**	Notes:

ILIOTIBIAL BAND (IT Band) - FOAM ROLL

Lie on your side with a foam roll under your bottom thigh. Use your arms and unaffected leg and then roll up and down the foam roll along the outside of your thigh.

ILIOTIBIAL BAND (IT Band) - BALL

Lie on your side or sit in chair. Hold small ball and move along the outside of the thigh.   Hold on the target muscle.

	_____ Reps _____ Sets _____X Day _____Hold		_____ Reps _____ Sets _____X Day _____Hold
23	Notes:	**24**	Notes:

PLANTAR FASCIA ROLLING – BALL

Sit and place ball under foot. Roll plantar fascia over ball back and forth.

PLANTAR FASCIA ROLLING - COLD SODA CAN

Sit and place cold soda can under foot. Roll plantar fascia over can back and forth.

Flexibility (Stretching)

Range of motion within a joint across various planes of motion that can be increased with stretching. This is needed to prevent decreased range of motion in a joint. Joint mobility can be inhibited by body habitués, genetics, connective tissue elasticity, skin that surrounds the joint, or the joint itself.

Some of the benefits of stretching: *(ACE Personal Training Manual)*	• Increased physical efficiency and performance. • Decreased risk of injury by decreasing resistance in various tissues. • Increased blood supply and nutrients to joint structures. • Improved nutrient exchange by increasing the quantity and decreasing the thickness of synovial fluid in the joint. • Increased neuromuscular coordination. • Improved muscular balance and postural awareness. • Reduced muscular tension. *(Bryant & Daniel, Ace Personal Training Manual, 2003, pg 306-307)*
Things to remember when stretching	• It is always better to stretch a warm muscle (*see Warm up and Cool down*) when the tissue temperature is above normal. Think of putting an elastic band in the freezer compared to heating it before stretching. Which do you think will get a better stretch? • Static stretching is best for the type for beginning athletes. Static stretching is a slow, gradual lengthening of the connective tissue (tendon, muscles and ligaments) through a full range of motion to the point of discomfort – not pain. This stretch should be held for at least 30 seconds, but no longer than two minutes. • Dynamic stretching consists of controlled leg and arm swings that take you to the limits of your range of motion. This type of stretching is appropriate to perform part of a warmup and/or cool down. • Ballistic stretching is a rapid, bouncing movement that may be appropriate in some sports. The problem is that there is also a high-risk factor for injury and should only be done with a professional's guidance. • Again, always remember to warm up before stretching. Repeat all stretches 2-3 times and hold for 15-30 seconds up to 60 seconds) unless otherwise indicated. • Some evidence shows that static stretching may be more beneficial at the end of the exercise program when there is more certainty that the muscles have warmed up. • Dynamic stretching may be more beneficial at the beginning of the exercise program as part of your warmup. This can also be done at the end as part of the cool down.

EXERCISE Flexibility (Stretching)	EXERCISE NUMBER	NOTES
INVERSION	1	
EVERSION	2	
ANTERIOR TIBIALIS	3	
PLANTARFLEXION	4	
DORSIFLEXION - STRAP	5	
DORSIFLEXION - FLOOR ASSISTED	6	
STANDING CALF STRETCH - GASTROC	7	
STANDING CALF STRETCH - GASTROC – HAND ON KNEE	8	
GASTROCNEMIUS STAIR STRETCH	9	
STANDING CALF STRETCH - SOLEUS	10	
HAMSTRING STRETCH – TOWEL, BAND, STRAP or BELT	11	
HAMSTRING STRETCH – TOWEL, BAND, STRAP or BELT	12	
HAMSTRING STRETCH - TABLE, BED OR COUCH	13	
HAMSTRING / KNEE EXTENSION STRETCH - SEATED	14	
HAMSTRING STRETCH - STANDING	15	
TOE TOUCH – STANDING - NARROW or WIDE BOS	16	
HEEL SLIDES - SELF ASSISTED	17	
HEEL SLIDES - LONG SIT ASSISTED - TOWEL, BAND, STRAP or BELT	18	
HEEL SLIDES - SUPINE	19	
KNEE BENDS - EXERCISE BALL	20	
KNEE FLEXION – SELF ASSISTED - PRONE	21	
KNEE FLEXION – BELT ASSISTED - PRONE	22	
HEEL SLIDES - SELF ASSISTED	23	
HEEL SLIDES - SEATED	24	
KNEE FLEXION – SCOOT FORWARD - SEATED	25	

Flexibility (Stretching)

EXERCISE Flexibility (Stretching)	EXERCISE NUMBER	NOTES
KNEE FLEXION – STAIR OR STEP	26	
PIRIFORMIS STRETCH	27	
PIRIFORMIS STRETCH - EXERCISE BALL	28	
PIRIFORMIS STRETCH - LONG SIT	29	
PIRIFORMIS STRETCH – STANDING	30	
HIP FLEXOR STRETCH - SIDE OF BALL or CHAIR	31	
HIP FLEXOR STRETCH - STANDING	32	
HIP FLEXOR STRETCH - HALF KNEEL	33	
RUNNER'S STRETCH - MODIFIED	34	
HIP FLEXOR STRETCH – SUPINE	35	
HIP FLEXOR STRETCH – SUPINE - 2	36	
QUAD STRETCH - SIDELYING	37	
QUAD STRETCH - STANDING	38	
KNEE FALL OUT STRETCH or FROG STRETCH	39	
BUTTERFLY STRETCH	40	
HIP ADDUCTOR STRECH – KNEELING	41	
HIP ADDUCTOR STRECH - STANDING	42	
HIP EXTERNAL ROTATION STRETCH - SUPINE	43	
HIP INTERNAL ROTATION STRETCH - SEATED	44	
IT BAND STRETCH - STANDING	45	
IT BAND STRETCH -- SIDELYING	46	
NECK ROTATION and SIDE BENDS	47	
NECK FLEXION AND EXTENSION	48	
TRUNK FLEXION - SEATED	49	
LOW BACK STRETCH - SEATED	50	
LOW BACK STRETCH – STANDING - STRAIGHT & LATERAL	51	
LOW BACK STRETCH – RAIL OR DOORKNOB	52	

Flexibility (Stretching)

EXERCISE Flexibility (Stretching)	EXERCISE NUMBER	NOTES
PRAYER STRETCH and LATERAL	53	
PRAYER STRETCH - EXERCISE BALL	54	
CAT AND CAMEL	55	
KNEE TO CHEST STRETCH - SINGLE and BILATERAL	56	
PRONE ON ELBOWS	57	
PRESS UPS	58	
TRUNK ROTATION STRETCH – SINGLE LEG	59	
LOWER TRUNK ROTATIONS – BILATERAL	60	
TRUNK ROTATION - SEATED	61	
TRUNK ROTATION - STANDING or SEATED – DOWEL	62	
LATERAL TRUNK STRETCH - SINGLE, SEATED or STANDING	63	
LATERAL TRUNK STRETCH - BILATERAL SEATED or STANDING	64	
FLEXION - SUPINE - DOWEL	65	
WALL WALK	66	
FLEXION - TABLE SLIDE	67	
FLEXION - TABLE SLIDE - BALL	68	
EXTERNAL ROTATION - SUPINE – DOWEL *INTERNAL ROTATION ON OPPOSITE ARM*	69	
EXTERNAL ROTATION - 90-90 - DOWEL	70	
EXTERNAL ROTATION – SEATED – DOWEL *INTERNAL ROTATION ON OPPOSITE ARM*	71	
EXTERNAL ROTATION – STANDING – DOWEL *INTERNAL ROTATION ON OPPOSITE ARM*	72	
ABDUCTION - TABLE SLIDE - BALL	75	
ABDUCTION WITH DOWEL	76	
LYING DOWN EXTENSION - TABLE or BED	77	
WAND EXTENSION - STANDING	78	
CHEST STRETCH – SEATED, STANDING, or SUPINE	79	

Flexibility (Stretching)

EXERCISE Flexibility (Stretching)	EXERCISE NUMBER	NOTES
TRICEP STRETCH - STRAP or TOWEL	82	
POSTERIOR SHOULDER/DELTOID RELEASE	83	
POSTERIOR CAPSULE STRETCH	84	

Stretching / Range of Motion (ROM)

Inversion

	_____ Reps _____ Sets _____ X Day _____ Hold
1	**Notes:**

INVERSION

Sit and cross your legs so that the target leg is on top. Hold your foot and pull upwards until a stretch is felt along the side of your ankle.

Eversion

	_____ Reps _____ Sets _____ X Day _____ Hold
2	**Notes:**

EVERSION

Sit and cross your legs so that the target leg is on top. Hold your foot and push downward until a stretch is felt along the inner side of your ankle.

Anterior Tibialis (Ant Tib)

	_____ Reps _____ Sets _____ X Day _____ Hold
3	**Notes:**

ANTERIOR TIBIALIS

Kneel upright and slowly sit back onto legs forcing heels down towards floor. Sit back until stretch is felt.

Plantarflexion (PF) *DF not shown*

	_____ Reps _____ Sets _____ X Day _____ Hold
4	**Notes:**

PLANTARFLEXION

Sit and place your affected foot on a firm surface. Use one hand bend the ankle downward as shown.

DORSIFLEXION – *Not shown*
Sit and place your affected foot on a firm surface. Use one hand under foot to push up towards shin (see #5 for movement)

Dorsiflexion (DF)

	_____ Reps _____ Sets _____X Day _____Hold		_____ Reps _____ Sets _____X Day _____Hold
5	**Notes:**	**6**	**Notes:**

DORSIFLEXION - STRAP

Sit with heel on floor and leg straight. Place belt/strap on forefoot and pull back until stretch is felt.

DORSIFLEXION - FLOOR ASSISTED

Sit and slide your foot back towards under the chair until a stretch is felt at the ankle.

Gastroc/Soleus

	_____ Reps _____ Sets _____X Day _____Hold		_____ Reps _____ Sets _____X Day _____Hold
7	**Notes:**	**8**	**Notes:**

Target Leg

STANDING CALF STRETCH - GASTROC

Stand in front of a wall, chair, or other sturdy object. Step forward with one foot and maintain your toes on both feet to be pointed straight forward. Keep the leg behind you with a straight knee during the stretch. Lean forward as you allow your front knee to bend until a stretch is felt along the back of your leg. Move closer or further away from the wall to control the stretch of the back leg.

Target Leg

STANDING CALF STRETCH - GASTROC – HAND ON KNEE

Step forward with one foot and place hand on thigh. Maintain your toes on both feet to be pointed straight forward. Keep the leg behind you with a straight knee during the stretch. Lean forward as you allow your front knee to bend until a stretch is felt along the back of your leg. You can adjust the bend of the front knee to control the stretch.

	_____ Reps _____ Sets _____X Day _____Hold		_____ Reps _____ Sets _____X Day _____Hold
9	Notes:	**10**	Notes:

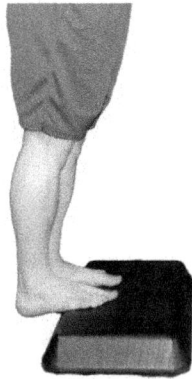

GASTROCNEMIUS STAIR STRETCH

Stand with the middle of your foot on the edge of the stairs while holding onto the railing. Slowly drop heels off until you feel a stretch in the back of your legs keeping your knees straight.

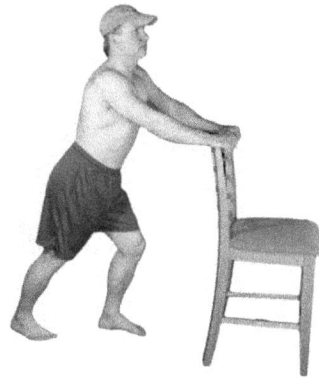

STANDING CALF STRETCH - SOLEUS

Stand in front of a wall, chair or other sturdy object. Step forward with one foot and maintain your toes on both feet to be pointed straight forward. Keep the leg behind you with a slightly bent knee during the stretch. Lean forward towards the wall and support yourself with your arms as you allow your front knee to bend until a gentle stretch is felt along the back of your leg. *Move closer or further away from the wall to control the stretch of the back leg. You can also adjust the bend of the front knee to control the stretch.

Hamstring / Knee Extension

	_____ Reps _____ Sets _____X Day _____Hold		_____ Reps _____ Sets _____X Day _____Hold
11	Notes:	**12**	Notes:

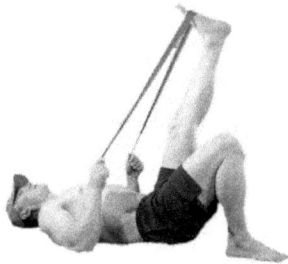

HAMSTRING STRETCH – TOWEL, BAND, STRAP or BELT

Lie down on your back and hook a towel/strap under your foot and draw up your leg until a stretch is felt under your leg/calf area. Keep your knee in a straightened position during the stretch. To increase stretch move strap to forefoot and flex foot.

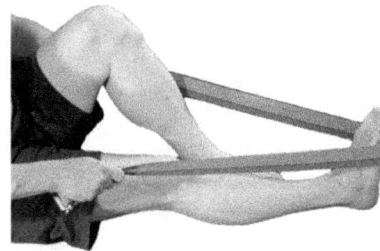

HAMSTRING STRETCH – TOWEL, BAND, STRAP or BELT

While pushing down on thigh above knee cap with opposite hand, pull on towel/ strap to lift heel from floor. Keep thigh flat. To increase stretch move strap to forefoot and flex foot and/or lean forward at the hip.

	_____ Reps _____ Sets _____X Day _____Hold
13	Notes:

HAMSTRING STRETCH - TABLE, BED OR COUCH

Sit on a raised flat surface where you can prop your target leg up on it such as a treatment table, couch or bed. While keeping your knee straight, slowly lean forward and reach your hands towards your foot until a gentle stretch is felt along the back of your knee/thigh. Hold and then return to starting position and repeat. Allow gravity to stretch your knee towards a more straightened position.
* Can use strap, towel or belt around forefoot as in #12

	_____ Reps _____ Sets _____X Day _____Hold
14	Notes:

HAMSTRING / KNEE EXTENSION STRETCH - SEATED

Sit and tighten your top thigh muscle to press the back of your knee downward towards the ground. You should feel a gentle stretch in the back of your knee.

* To increase stretch put strap to forefoot, flex foot and lean forward at the hip.

	_____ Reps _____ Sets _____X Day _____Hold
15	Notes:

HAMSTRING STRETCH - STANDING

Stand and rest your foot on a stool/box/step with your knee straight. Gently lean forward at the hips until a stretch is felt behind your knee/thigh. Keep your back straight. *To increase stretch, flex your foot at the ankle, and/or put strap to forefoot and flex foot. If on stair, you can put foot on 2nd or 3rd step.

	_____ Reps _____ Sets _____X Day _____Hold
16	Notes:

TOE TOUCH – STANDING - NARROW or WIDE BOS

Stand and bend forward at waist keep legs straight and reach for toes. Can perform with either narrow or wide base of support.

Knee Flexion

_____Reps _____Sets _____X Day _____Hold	_____Reps _____Sets _____X Day _____Hold

17 Notes: **18** Notes:

HEEL SLIDES - SELF ASSISTED

Lie on your back with knees straight and slide the target heel towards your buttock as you bend your knee. Use the unaffected leg to assist the bending. Hold a gentle stretch in this position and then return to original position.

HEEL SLIDES - LONG SIT ASSISTED - TOWEL, BAND, STRAP or BELT

Sit with legs straight. Can place a small hand towel under your heel to help slide. Loop a band around your foot and pull your knee into a bend position as your foot slides towards your buttock. Hold a gentle stretch and then return back to original position.

_____Reps _____Sets _____X Day _____Hold	_____Reps _____Sets _____X Day _____Hold

19 Notes: **20** Notes:

HEEL SLIDES - SUPINE

Lie on your back with knees straight and slide the target heel towards your buttock as you bend your knee. Hold a gentle stretch in this position and then return to original position.

KNEE BENDS - EXERCISE BALL

Lie on your back and place your heels on an exercise ball. Roll it closer to your buttocks as your knees and hips bend as shown. Hold and then return to original position. *If you have limited range in one knee, use the other leg to help increase range of motion.

Flexibility (Stretching)

	_____ Reps _____ Sets _____ X Day _____ Hold		_____ Reps _____ Sets _____ X Day _____ Hold
21	Notes:	**22**	Notes:

KNEE FLEXION – SELF ASSISTED - PRONE

Lie face down and bend your target knee with the assistance of your unaffected leg.

KNEE FLEXION – BELT ASSISTED - PRONE

Lie face down with a strap looped around your target side ankle or foot. Use the belt to pull the knee into a bent position allowing for a stretch.

	_____ Reps _____ Sets _____ X Day _____ Hold		_____ Reps _____ Sets _____ X Day _____ Hold
23	Notes:	**24**	Notes:

HEEL SLIDES - SELF ASSISTED

It and slide your heel towards your buttock with the assist of the unaffected leg. Hold a gentle stretch and then return foot forward to original position.

HEEL SLIDES - SEATED – can use towel or paper under foot to help slide

Sit and place your feet on the floor (can put target foot on a towel or paper to help slide if needed). Slowly slide your foot closer towards you. Hold a gentle stretch and then return foot forward to original position.

	_____ Reps _____ Sets _____X Day _____Hold		_____ Reps _____ Sets _____X Day _____Hold
25	Notes:	**26**	Notes:

Plant foot. Scoot hips forward.

KNEE FLEXION – SCOOT FORWARD - SEATED

Sit and slide your foot back to a bent knee position. Keep your foot planted on the ground and scoot forward until a stretch is felt at the knee. Hold the stretch and then scoot back to original position.

KNEE FLEXION – STAIR OR STEP

Place target foot on stool or step with bent knee. Gently bend forward keeping heel on step. Hold the stretch and then return to original position.

Piriformis

	_____ Reps _____ Sets _____X Day _____Hold		_____ Reps _____ Sets _____X Day _____Hold
27	Notes:	**28**	Notes:

PIRIFORMIS STRETCH

Lie on your back with both knees bent. Cross your target leg on the other knee. Hold your unaffected thigh and pull it up towards your chest until a stretch is felt in the buttock.

PIRIFORMIS STRETCH - EXERCISE BALL

Lie on your back with one foot placed on the ball. Cross your other leg over the knee of the leg on the ball and gently roll the ball back towards your chest until a stretch is felt in the buttock.

	_____ Reps _____ Sets _____X Day _____Hold		_____ Reps _____ Sets _____X Day _____Hold
29	Notes:	**30**	Notes:

PIRIFORMIS STRETCH - LONG SIT

Sit with one knee straight and the other bent and placed over the opposite knee. Gentle turn your body towards the bend knee side.

PIRIFORMIS STRETCH – STANDING

Stand with unaffected leg crossed in front of target side. Lean forward reaching for foot on target side until stretch is felt in the buttock.

Hip Flexors

	_____ Reps _____ Sets _____X Day _____Hold		_____ Reps _____ Sets _____X Day _____Hold
31	Notes:	**32**	Notes:

HIP FLEXOR STRETCH - SIDE OF BALL or CHAIR

Sit on edge of chair or ball. Bend your front knee (unaffected side) and lean forward until a stretch is felt along the front of the target hip.

HIP FLEXOR STRETCH - STANDING

Stand and bend one knee forward (unaffected side) and the other in back. Stand up straight leaning slightly backward until a stretch is felt along the front of the target hip.

_____ Reps _____ Sets _____ X Day _____ Hold		_____ Reps _____ Sets _____ X Day _____ Hold	
33	Notes:	**34**	Notes:

HIP FLEXOR STRETCH - HALF KNEEL – with or without pad under knee

Begin in a half-kneeling position (you may want to use a pad or pillow for cushion). Bend your front knee (unaffected side) and lean forward until a stretch is felt along the front of the target hip.

RUNNER'S STRETCH - MODIFIED

Stretch target leg in back and bend other knee in front. Bend your front knee (unaffected side) and lean forward until a stretch is felt along the front of the target hip.

_____ Reps _____ Sets _____ X Day _____ Hold		_____ Reps _____ Sets _____ X Day _____ Hold	
35	Notes:	**36**	Notes:

HIP FLEXOR STRETCH – SUPINE

Lie on a table, high bed or matt and let the affected leg lower towards the floor until a stretch is felt along the front of your thigh.

HIP FLEXOR STRETCH – SUPINE

Lie on a table, high bed or matt and let the affected leg lower towards the floor until a stretch is felt along the front of your thigh. At the same time, grasp your opposite knee and pull it towards your chest.

Quadriceps (Quad)

	_____ Reps _____ Sets _____ X Day _____ Hold		_____ Reps _____ Sets _____ X Day _____ Hold
37	Notes:	**38**	Notes:

QUAD STRETCH - SIDELYING

Lie on your side and reach back holding the top of your foot with bent knee until a stretch is felt.

QUAD STRETCH - STANDING

Stand straight up and bend your knee in back holding your ankle/foot. Gently pull your knee/thigh back in alignment with the standing leg.

Adductor

	_____ Reps _____ Sets _____ X Day _____ Hold		_____ Reps _____ Sets _____ X Day _____ Hold
39	Notes:	**40**	Notes:

One Leg

Both Legs

KNEE FALL OUT STRETCH or FROG STRETCH

Lie on your back with one knee bent. Slowly lower your knee to the side as you stretch the inner thigh/hip area. Frog Stretch: Let both knees fall to the side at the same time.

BUTTERFLY STRETCH

Sit on the floor or mat and bend your knees placing the bottom of your feet together. Slowly let your knees lower towards the floor until a stretch is felt at your inner thighs.

	_____ Reps _____ Sets _____X Day _____Hold		_____ Reps _____ Sets _____X Day _____Hold
41	**Notes:**	**42**	**Notes:**

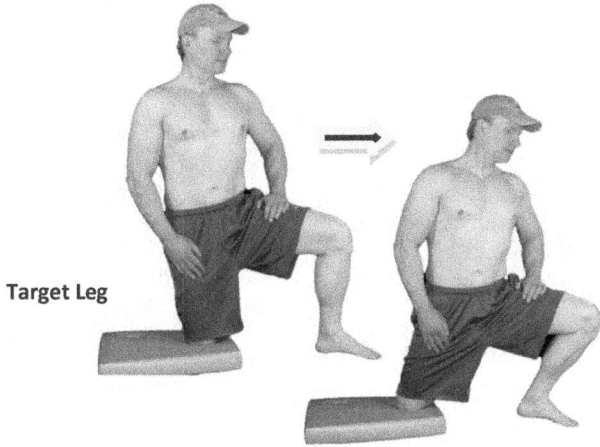

Target Leg

HIP ADDUCTOR STRECH – KNEELING

Kneel down on your target side knee. Place the opposite leg directly out to the side. Lean towards the side as you bend the knee for a stretch to the inner thigh of the target leg.

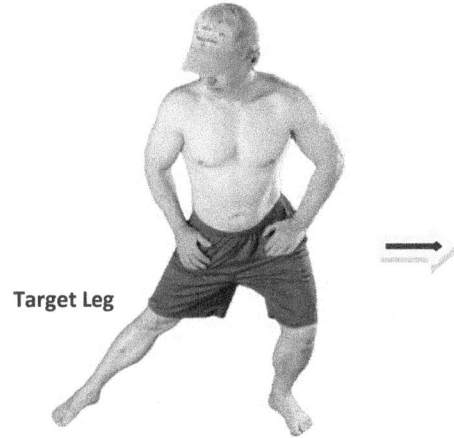

Target Leg

HIP ADDUCTOR STRECH - STANDING

Stand with feet spread wide apart. Slowly bend your knee to allow for a gentle stretch of the opposite leg. Maintain a straight knee on the target leg the entire time. You should feel a stretch on the inner thigh.

External Rotation / Internal Rotation

	_____ Reps _____ Sets _____X Day _____Hold		_____ Reps _____ Sets _____X Day _____Hold
43	**Notes:**	**44**	**Notes:**

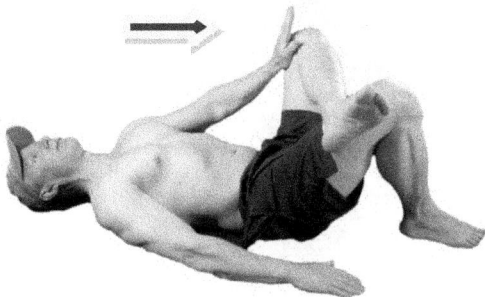

HIP EXTERNAL ROTATION STRETCH - SUPINE

Lie on your back with your leg crossed over your knee. Use your hand and push the crossed knee away from you.

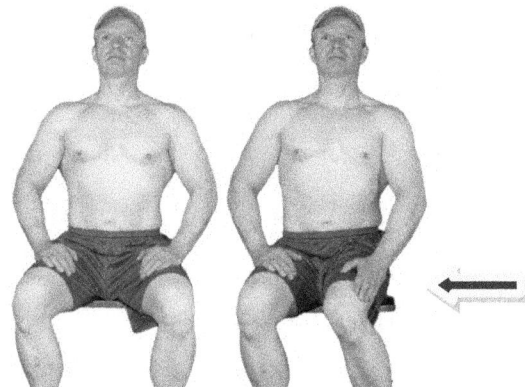

HIP INTERNAL ROTATION STRETCH - SEATED

Sit on a chair with your legs spread apart and feet planted on the ground. Use your hand to draw your knee inward as shown.

Iliotibial Band (IT Band)

	_____ Reps _____ Sets _____ X Day _____ Hold

45 | Notes:

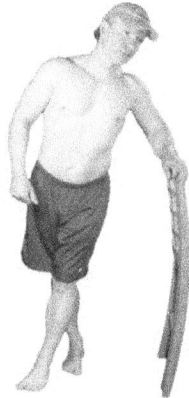

IT BAND STRETCH - STANDING

Stand and cross the target leg behind your unaffected leg. Lean forward and towards the unaffected side while using your arm for balance support.

	_____ Reps _____ Sets _____ X Day _____ Hold

46 | Notes:

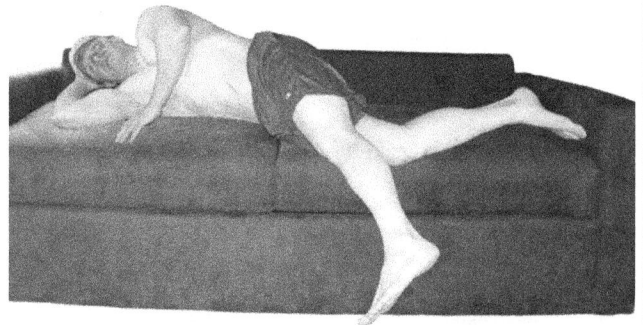

IT BAND STRETCH -- SIDELYING

Lie on bed or couch on unaffected side with target side towards ceiling. Bend lower leg for support. Allow upper leg to drop over side of bed. Keep knee straight and point toe towards floor. May need to roll upper hip backwards in order to feel stretch on side of hip/thigh/knee.

NECK

	_____ Reps _____ Sets _____ X Day _____ Hold

47 | Notes:

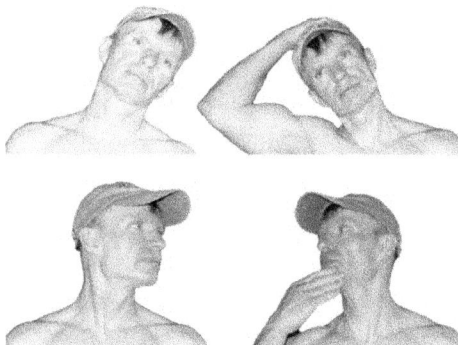

NECK ROTATION and SIDE BENDS

SIDE BENDS: (_Top_) Tilt your head as if you are trying to touch your ear to your shoulder. For extra stretch gently use your hand to increase range and hold.
ROTATION: (_Bottom_) Turn your head to the side as if looking over your shoulder. For an extra stretch gently use your hand on your chin to increase range and hold.

	_____ Reps _____ Sets _____ X Day _____ Hold

48 | Notes:

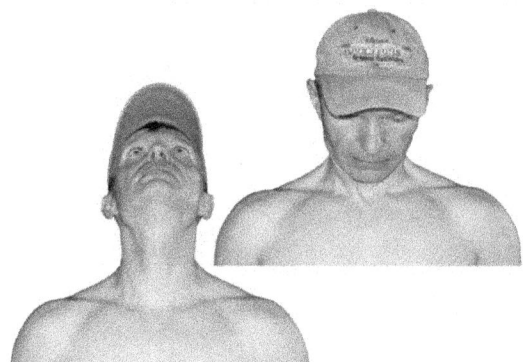

NECK FLEXION AND EXTENSION

EXTENSION: Look up as if you are looking at the sky moving your neck only.
FLEXION: Look down as if you are looking at the floor. For an extra stretch gently put both hands behind your head to move chin towards the chest and hold.

BACK

_____ Reps _____ Sets _____ X Day _____ Hold		_____ Reps _____ Sets _____ X Day _____ Hold	
49	Notes:	**50**	Notes:

TRUNK FLEXION - SEATED

Sit and cross your arms over your chest. Slowly curl your back forward in order to round your upper back.

LOW BACK STRETCH - SEATED

Sit and slowly bend forward reaching your hands for the floor. Bend your trunk and head forward and down.

_____ Reps _____ Sets _____ X Day _____ Hold		_____ Reps _____ Sets _____ X Day _____ Hold	
51	Notes:	**52**	Notes:

LOW BACK STRETCH – STANDING - STRAIGHT & LATERAL

Stand in front of a table / chair or other surface and bend forward at the waist. Support yourself with your hands on a surface.

Reach to the side for a lateral bend (see #53)

LOW BACK STRETCH – RAIL OR DOORKNOB

Hold onto doorknob, rail or other unmovable surface and pull while moving hips back and hold.

_____ Reps _____ Sets _____ X Day _____ Hold

53 | **Notes:**

Lateral

Straight

PRAYER STRETCH and LATERAL

STRAIGHT: Start on your hands and knees. Slowly lower your buttocks towards your feet until a stretch is felt along your back and or buttocks.

LATERAL: Start on your hands and knees. Slowly lower your buttocks towards your feet. Lower your chest towards the floor as you reach out towards the side.

_____ Reps _____ Sets _____X Day _____Hold

54 | **Notes:**

PRAYER STRETCH - EXERCISE BALL

Kneel with an exercise ball in front of you. Slowly lean forward and roll the ball forward until a stretch is felt.

*Can do lateral movement as in #53

_____ Reps _____ Sets _____X Day _____Hold

55 | **Notes:**

CAT AND CAMEL

Start on your hands and knees. Raise up your back and arch it towards the ceiling (cat). Return to a lowered position and arch your back the opposite direction (camel).

_____ Reps _____ Sets _____X Day _____Hold

56 | **Notes:**

Both Legs

One Leg

KNEE TO CHEST STRETCH - SINGLE and BILATERAL

BILATERAL: Lie on your back and hold your knees while pulling up towards your chest and hold.
SINGLE: Lie on your back and hold your knee while pulling up towards your chest and hold. Opposite leg can be straight or bent.

Trunk Extension

	_____ Reps _____ Sets _____X Day _____Hold		_____ Reps _____ Sets _____X Day _____Hold
57	**Notes:**	**58**	**Notes:**

PRONE ON ELBOWS

Lie on your stomach. Slowly press up and prop yourself up on your elbows. Keep hips on floor/mat.

PRESS UPS

Lie on your stomach. Slowly press up and arch your back using your arms. Keep hips on floor/mat.

Trunk Rotation

	_____ Reps _____ Sets _____X Day _____Hold		_____ Reps _____ Sets _____X Day _____Hold
59	**Notes:**	**60**	**Notes:**

TRUNK ROTATION STRETCH – SINGLE LEG

Lie on your back with arms to the sides. Bend one knee and then raise it up and across your body. Allow your trunk to rotate for a gentle stretch to the spine. Hold and then repeat.

LOWER TRUNK ROTATIONS – BILATERAL

Lie on your back with your knees bent and gently move your knees side-to-side.

_____ Reps _____ Sets _____ X Day _____ Hold		_____ Reps _____ Sets _____ X Day _____ Hold
61 Notes:	**62**	Notes:

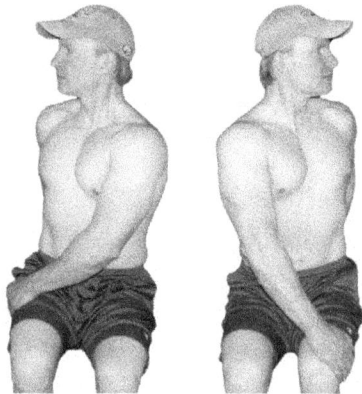

TRUNK ROTATION - SEATED

Sit up as tall with erect posture. Rotate in one direction, using your hand to press against the opposite thigh to aide in further rotation. Exhale to increase the rotation and stretch. Return to the starting position, maintain an upright posture -repeat in the opposite direction.

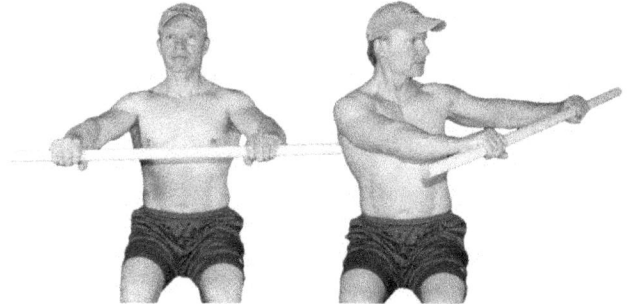

TRUNK ROTATION - STANDING or SEATED – DOWEL

Stand or sit holding dowel in hands. Slowly rotate trunk in one direction and then in the opposite direction.

Lateral

_____ Reps _____ Sets _____ X Day _____ Hold		_____ Reps _____ Sets _____ X Day _____ Hold
63 Notes:	**64**	Notes:

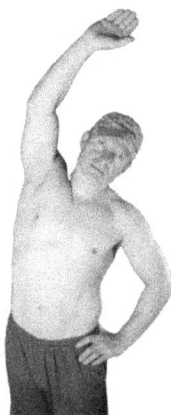

LATERAL TRUNK STRETCH - SINGLE
SEATED or STANDING

Raise your arm and bend to the opposite side for a stretch. Hold and repeat with opposite arm.

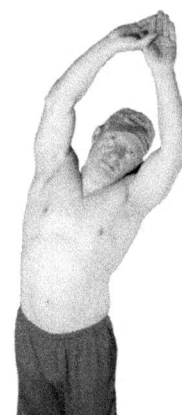

LATERAL TRUNK STRETCH - BILATERAL
SEATED or STANDING

Clasp hands together and raise arms over head. Bend to one side. Hold and repeat in opposite direction.

Shoulder Flexion

	_____Reps _____Sets _____X Day _____Hold		_____Reps _____Sets _____X Day _____Hold
65	Notes:	66	Notes:

FLEXION - SUPINE - DOWEL

Lie on your back and hold a dowel/cane. Slowly raise the dowel overhead.

*If you have a weak or injured arm, you can use your unaffected arm to assist with the movement.

WALL WALK

Place your target hand on the wall with the palm facing the wall. Walk your fingers up the wall towards overhead. Slide or walk your hand back down the wall to the starting position.

	_____Reps _____Sets _____X Day _____Hold		_____Reps _____Sets _____X Day _____Hold
67	Notes:	68	Notes:

FLEXION - TABLE SLIDE

Sit or stand and rest your target arm on a table and gently slide it forward and then back.

FLEXION - TABLE SLIDE - BALL

Stand and rest your target arm on top of a ball on a table. Gently roll the ball forward and then back.

Shoulder External Rotation (ER)

	_____ Reps _____ Sets _____ X Day _____ Hold		_____ Reps _____ Sets _____ X Day _____ Hold
69	Notes:	**70**	Notes:

Starting Position

EXTERNAL ROTATION - SUPINE – DOWEL
INTERNAL ROTATION ON OPPOSITE ARM

Lie on your back holding a dowel/cane with both hands. On the target side, maintain approx. 90-degree bend at the elbow with your arm approximately 30-45 degrees away from your side. Use your other arm to push the dowel/cane to rotate the affected arm back into a stretch. Hold and then return to starting position. Repeat

EXTERNAL ROTATION - 90-90 - DOWEL

Lie on your back and hold a dowel with your elbows out to the side and rested down. Roll your arms back towards overhead until a stretch is felt. Keep elbows bent at a 90-degree angle.

	_____ Reps _____ Sets _____ X Day _____ Hold		_____ Reps _____ Sets _____ X Day _____ Hold
71	Notes:	**72**	Notes:

EXTERNAL ROTATION – SEATED – DOWEL
INTERNAL ROTATION ON OPPOSITE ARM

Using the unaffected arm, push the dowel into the hand of the target arm. Keep the arm at a 90-degree angle and push until a stretch is felt. Hold and repeat.

EXTERNAL ROTATION – STANDING – DOWEL
INTERNAL ROTATION ON OPPOSITE ARM

Using the unaffected arm, push the dowel into the hand of the target arm. Keep the arm at a 90-degree angle and push until a stretch is felt. Hold and repeat.

Shoulder Internal Rotation (IR) - *also see #69, 71, 72*

	_____ Reps _____ Sets _____ X Day _____ Hold		_____ Reps _____ Sets _____ X Day _____ Hold
73	Notes:	**74**	Notes:

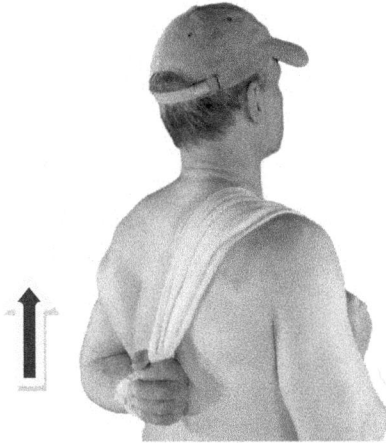

INTERNAL ROTATION – TOWEL OR STRAP

Hold one end of the towel in front and with the target arm behind your back. Gently pull up your target arm behind your back with the assist of a towel.

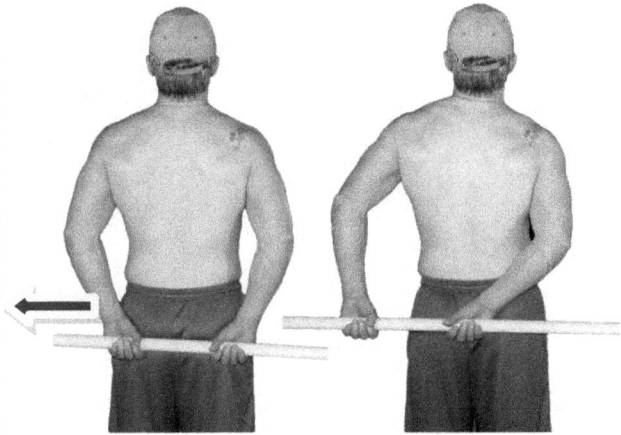

INTERNAL ROTATION – DOWEL

Hold a dowel/cane behind your back. Slowly pull the target arm towards the center of your back.

Shoulder Abduction

	_____ Reps _____ Sets _____ X Day _____ Hold		_____ Reps _____ Sets _____ X Day _____ Hold
75	Notes:	**76**	Notes:

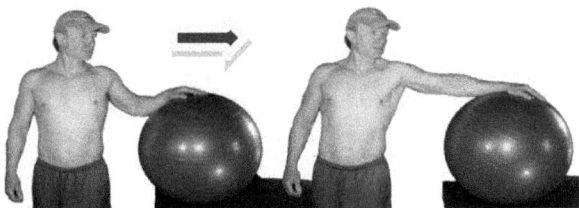

ABDUCTION - TABLE SLIDE - BALL

Stand and rest your target arm on top of a ball on a table and gently roll it to the side and back.

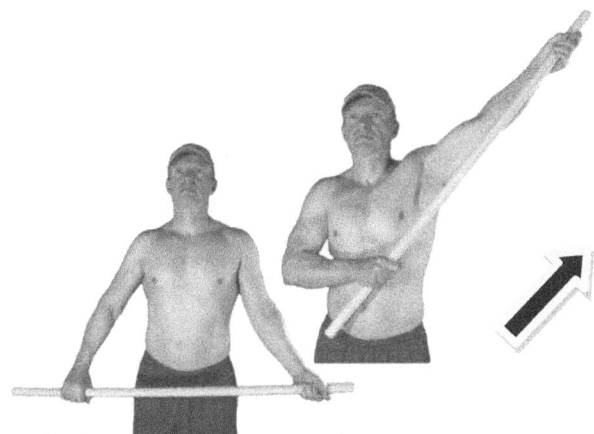

ABDUCTION WITH DOWEL

Hold a dowel/cane in front. Slowly push the dowel of the unaffected arm towards the target arm upward and to the side.

Shoulder Extension

	_____ Reps _____ Sets _____ X Day _____ Hold		_____ Reps _____ Sets _____ X Day _____ Hold
77	**Notes:**	**78**	**Notes:**

LYING DOWN EXTENSION - TABLE or BED

Lie on your back and gently let target arm drop off table or bed.

WAND EXTENSION - STANDING

Stand and hold a dowel/cane. Use the unaffected arm to help push the target arm back. The elbow should remain straight the entire time.

Chest/Pec Stretch

	_____ Reps _____ Sets _____ X Day _____ Hold		_____ Reps _____ Sets _____ X Day _____ Hold
79	**Notes:**	**80**	**Notes:**

CHEST STRETCH – SEATED, STANDING, or SUPINE

TOP: Bend arms at a 90-degree angle. Move elbows back until feeling a stretch in front of shoulders/chest.

BOTTOM: Clasp hands in back of head. Move elbows back until feeling a stretch in front of shoulders/chest.

CHEST STRETCH - STEP THROUGH

Stand with arms in doorway at a 90-degree angle. Step through until you feel a stretch through the chest and hold. Keep shoulders down and back. Take another step to increase stretch.

Triceps

	_____ Reps _____ Sets _____X Day _____Hold		_____ Reps _____ Sets _____X Day _____Hold
81	Notes:	82	Notes:

TRICEP STRETCH

With your target elbow bent and shoulder raised, use your other hand and gently push your target elbow back towards overhead until a stretch is felt.

TRICEP STRETCH - STRAP or TOWEL

Hold strap of target arm with your hand above your head. Use the other hand to pull downward on the strap, allowing the elbow to bend until a stretch is in the back of the arm.

Posterior Capsule

	_____ Reps _____ Sets _____X Day _____Hold		_____ Reps _____ Sets _____X Day _____Hold
83	Notes:	84	Notes:

POSTERIOR SHOULDER/DELTOID RELEASE

Bring your target arm across your body. Use the opposite hand to grasp the back of your shoulder and further pull the arm. Hold.

POSTERIOR CAPSULE STRETCH

Lie on your side and grasp the elbow of the arm closest to the floor. Gently pull it upward and across the front of your body.

Core / Stability Training

Core strengthening is the foundation of all the other exercises that follow, especially balance. Core training is not only an important step in conditioning, but also helps other issues, including neurological, orthopedic, weight, or overall weakness

The core includes muscles of the thoraco-lumbar spine (trunk), cervical spine., erector spinae, abdomen, pelvis, shoulder/scapulae, and your lower lats.

Static core functionality is the ability of one's core to align the skeleton to resist a force that does not change. The core is used to stabilize the thorax and the pelvis during dynamic movement. The nature of dynamic movement must consider our skeletal structure (as a lever) in addition to the force of external resistance and consequently incorporates a vastly different complex of muscles and joints versus a static position.

The core is traditionally assumed to originate most full-body functional movement, including most sports. In addition, the core determines to a large part a person's posture. In all, human anatomy is built to take force upon the bones and direct autonomic force, through various joints, in the desired direction. The core muscles align the spine, ribs, and pelvis of a person to resist a specific force, whether static or dynamic.
(Wikipedia: *https://en.wikipedia.org/wiki/Core_(anatomy)*)

These muscles work as stabilizers for the entire body. Core training is simply doing specific exercises to develop and strengthen these stabilizer muscles. If any of these core muscles are weakened, it could result in lower back pain or a protruding waistline. Keeping these core muscles strong can do wonders for your posture and help give you more strength in other exercises like running and walking.
(Bodybuilding.com - *https://www.bodybuilding.com/fun/mielke12.htm*)

There is a saying 'form follows function'. This is especially true with core stability and how it affects your balance. Gravity influences all movement, so effective core training must be done against gravity. The rectus abdominus muscle that you are isolating with those crunches flexes the spine/abs only when you are lying on your back or returning the torso to an upright position from hyperextension in standing. "In the upright position, flexion is controlled by eccentric contraction of the back extensors as the lower the weight of the torso in the same direction as gravity". (*Bryant & Green, 2003, p. 84*)

Being able to engage the core with not only your balance exercises but also arm and leg exercises will help prevent injury.

Step 1: First learn to brace the abdomen *(see pictures 1 and 2 on next page)* Think of this as trying to either brace for a punch to the stomach or trying to put on a tight pair of pants (not just sucking in your stomach)

Step 2: After getting a good feel for bracing, try doing a pelvic tilt *(see pictures 3 and 4 on next page)* and then progress to bridging *(see picture 5)*

Step 3: These two basic movements should be done while you progress your abdominal and core training, continuing through the balance section, and to some extent with arm and leg strengthening.

*** **When doing floor work, such as crunches, make sure you are on a soft surface, such as a mat, Bosu, stability ball, etc. Pushing your back into a hard surface, such as a wood floor, can do more damage than good to the spine.**

*** **Breathe – Never hold your breath.**

EXERCISE Core / Stability	EXERCISE NUMBER	NOTES
ABDOMINAL BRACING TRAINING	1	
ABDOMINAL BRACING - SUPINE	2	
PELVIC TILT - SUPINE	3	
PELVIC TILT - KNEELING	4	
BRIDGING	5	
BRIDGE - BOSU	6	
BRIDGING WITH PILLOW SQUEEZE	7	
BRIDGING WITH PILLOW SQUEEZE - BOSU	8	
BRACE SUPINE MARCHING / BRIDGE LEG UP	9	
BRIDGE LEG UP - BOSU -	10	
SINGLE LEG BRIDGE	11	
BRIDGE SINGLE LEG - BOSU	12	
BRIDGING CROSSED LEG	13	
BRIDGING CROSSED LEG – BOSU	14	
BRIDGING CROSSED LEG - ARMS UP	15	
BRIDGING CROSSED LEG - ARMS UP - BOSU	16	
BRIDGE - ELASTIC BAND	17	
BRIDGING - ABDUCTION - ELASTIC BAND	18	
FLOOR BRIDGE - EXERCISE BALL	19	
FLOOR BRIDGE ALTERNATE LEG LIFT - EXERCISE BALL	20	
BRIDGE UPPER BACK - EXERCISE BALL	21	
BRIDGE UPPER BACK - SINGLE LEG - EXERCISE BALL	22	
QUADRUPED ALTERNATE ARM	23	
QUADRUPED ALTERNATE LEG	24	
QUADRUPED ALTERNATE ARM AND LEG	25	
BIRD DOG ELBOW TOUCHES	26	

EXERCISE	EXERCISE NUMBER	NOTES
Core / Stability		
PRONE BALL	27	
PRONE BALL - ALTERNATE ARM	28	
PRONE BALL - ALTERNATE LEG	29	
PRONE BALL - ALTERNATE ARM AND LEG	30	
MODIFIED PLANK	31	
MODIFIED PLANK - ALTERNATE LEG	32	
FULL PLANK	33	
PLANK - ALTERNATE ARMS	34	
PLANK - ALTERNATE LEGS	35	
PLANK - EXERCISE BALL	36	
PRONE ON ELBOWS	37	
PRESS UPS	38	
SKYDIVER	39	
PRONE SUPERMAN - BOSU	40	
TRUNK EXTENSION - BOSU	41	
TRUNK EXTENSION - HANDS CROSSED IN FRONT - BOSU	43	
SUPERMAN - ARMS BACK- EXERCISE BALL	44	
SUPERMAN – BOTH ARMS IN FRONT - EXERCISE BALL	45	
SUPERMAN – ONE ARM FORWARD / ONE ARM BACK - EXERCISE BALL	46	
LATERAL PLANK MODIFIED	47	
LATERAL PLANK MODIFIED- BOSU	48	
LATERAL PLANK - 1 KNEE 1 FOOT	49	
LATERAL PLANK - 1 KNEE 1 FOOT – BOSU	50	
LATERAL PLANK	51	
LATERAL PLANK - BOSU	52	

EXERCISE Core / Stability	EXERCISE NUMBER	NOTES
LEAN BACK	53	
LEAN BACK - BOSU	54	
LEAN BACK WITH ARMS OUT	55	
LEAN BACK WITH ARMS OUT - BOSU	56	
LEAN BACK WITH TWIST	57	
LEAN BACK WITH TWIST – BOSU	58	
CRUNCHY FROG	59	
SEATED BIKE - FORWARD AND BACKWARDS	60	
CRUNCH – ARMS OUT	61	
CRUNCH – ARMS OUT - BOSU	62	
CRUNCH – ARMS IN BACK OF HEAD	63	
CRUNCH – ARMS IN BACK OF HEAD - BOSU	64	
OBLIQUE CRUNCH	65	
OBLIQUE CRUNCH - BOSU	66	
90 DEGREE CRUNCH	67	
BALL CRUNCH – Can put legs on seat of chair	68	
CURL UPS – ARMS ON LEGS - EXERCISE BALL	69	
CURL UPS- ARMS CROSSED IN FRONT - EXERCISE BALL	70	
CURL UPS – ARMS BEHIND HEAD - EXERCISE BALL	71	
SUPINE CRUNCH TOUCH - EXERCISE BALL	72	
LOWER ABDOMINAL CRUNCH – WITH or WITHOUT BALL	73	
HIGH MARCH CRUNCH	74	
STANDING SIDE CRUNCH	75	
STANDING BIKE CRUNCH	76	

Core/Abdominal

Abdominal Bracing – Pelvic Tilt

1	_____ Reps _____ Sets _____X Day _____Hold **Notes:**	

ABDOMINAL BRACING TRAINING

Press your fingertips into your relaxed abdomen lateral of your navel. Tighten and brace your abdomen so that the muscles push your fingertips away from the center of your body. Hold, relax and repeat.
Think of this as trying to either brace for a punch to the stomach or trying to put on a tight pair of pants (not just sucking in your stomach)

2	_____ Reps _____ Sets _____X Day _____Hold **Notes:**	

Starting Position

ABDOMINAL BRACING - SUPINE

Lie on your back. Tighten your stomach muscles as you draw your navel down towards the floor.

Think of this as trying to either brace for a punch to the stomach or trying to put on a tight pair of pants (not just sucking in your stomach)

3	_____ Reps _____ Sets _____X Day _____Hold **Notes:**	

Starting Position

PELVIC TILT - SUPINE

Lie on your back with your knees bent. Next, arch your low back and then flatten it repeatedly (bracing as above). Your pelvis should tilt forward and back during the movement. Move through a comfortable range of motion.

4	_____ Reps _____ Sets _____X Day _____Hold **Notes:**	

Starting Position

PELVIC TILT - KNEELING

Kneel on the floor (you can kneel on a pillow or pad if needed). Arch your lower back and then flatten it repeatedly (bracing as above). Your pelvis should tilt forward and back during the movement. Move through a comfortable range of motion.

Bridging	

_____ Reps _____ Sets _____X Day _____Hold	_____ Reps _____ Sets _____X Day _____Hold
5 Notes:	**6** Notes:

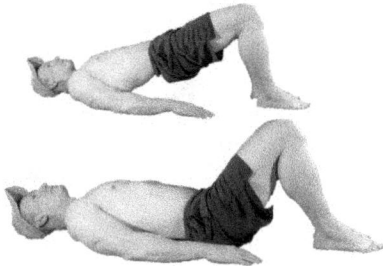

Starting

Position

BRIDGING

Lie on your back. Tighten your lower abdominals (as with abdominal bracing), squeeze your buttocks and then raise your buttocks off the floor/bed. Hold and then lower yourself slowly and repeat. Brace the stomach muscles to keep your spine from moving, trying to keep the pelvis level the entire time.

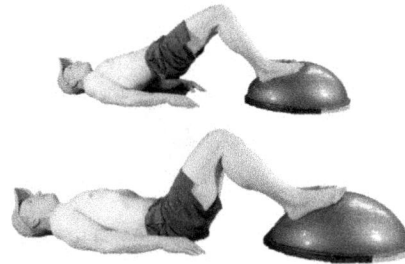

Starting
Position

BRIDGE - BOSU – Can use foam pad, stair step or box

Lie on your back with your feet planted on top of the Bosu and knees bent. Lift up your buttocks as shown. Hold and then lower yourself slowly and repeat.
Brace the stomach muscles to keep your spine from moving, trying to keep the pelvis level the entire time.

_____ Reps _____ Sets _____X Day _____Hold	_____ Reps _____ Sets _____X Day _____Hold
7 Notes:	**8** Notes:

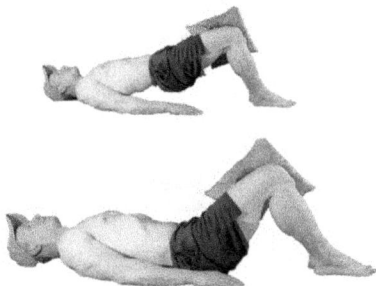

Starting

Position

BRIDGING WITH PILLOW SQUEEZE - Use pillow, ball or rolled towel between knees

Lie on your back and place a pillow, towel roll or ball between your knees and squeeze. Hold this and then tighten your lower abdominals, squeeze your buttocks and raise your buttocks off the floor/bed. Brace the stomach muscles to keep your spine from moving, trying to keep the pelvis level.

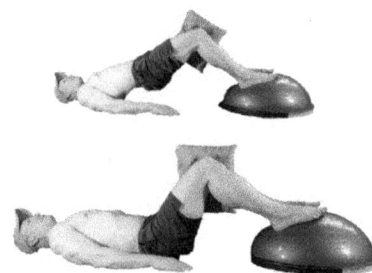

Starting

Position

BRIDGING WITH PILLOW SQUEEZE - BOSU - Can use foam pad, stair step or box

Lie on your back with your feet planted on top of the Bosu and knees bent. Place a pillow, towel roll or ball between your knees and squeeze. Lift up your buttocks as shown. Hold and then lower yourself slowly and repeat. Brace the stomach muscles to keep your spine from moving, trying to keep the pelvis level.

_____ Reps _____ Sets _____ X Day _____ Hold		_____ Reps _____ Sets _____ X Day _____ Hold	
9	Notes:	**10**	Notes:

Starting Position

BRACE SUPINE MARCHING / BRIDGE LEG UP

Lie on your back with your knees bent, slowly lift up one foot a few inches and then set it back down. Perform on your other leg. Brace the stomach muscles to keep your spine from moving, trying to keep the pelvis level the entire time.
*To increase challenge, go into bridge position as with #5, then continue march – can bring leg higher to advance

Starting Position

BRIDGE LEG UP - BOSU - Can use foam pad, stair step or box

Lie on your back with your feet planted on top of the Bosu and knees bent. Slowly lift up one foot a few inches and then set it back down. Next, perform on your other leg. Brace the stomach muscles to keep your spine from moving, trying to keep the pelvis level the entire time. *To increase challenge, go into bridge position as with #6, then continue march – can bring leg higher to advance

_____ Reps _____ Sets _____ X Day _____ Hold		_____ Reps _____ Sets _____ X Day _____ Hold	
11	Notes:	**12**	Notes:

Starting Position

SINGLE LEG BRIDGE

Lie on your back, raise your buttocks off the floor/bed into a bridge position. Straighten a leg so that only one leg is supporting your body. Then, return that leg back to the ground and change to the other side. Brace the stomach muscles to keep your spine from moving, trying to keep the pelvis level the entire time.

Starting Position

BRIDGE SINGLE LEG - BOSU - can use foam pad, stair step or box

Lie on your back with your feet planted on top of the Bosu and knees bent, lift up your buttocks and then straighten one knee in the air. Return that leg back to the ground and change to the other side. Brace the stomach muscles to keep your spine from moving, trying to keep the pelvis level the entire time.

_____ Reps _____ Sets _____ X Day _____ Hold		_____ Reps _____ Sets _____ X Day _____ Hold

13 | Notes: | **14** | Notes:

Starting
Position

BRIDGING CROSSED LEG

Lie on your back, cross your leg. Tighten your lower abdomen, squeeze your buttocks and raise your buttocks off the floor/bed. Brace the stomach muscles to keep your spine from moving, trying to keep the pelvis level the entire time.

Starting Position

BRIDGING CROSSED LEG – BOSU - can use foam pad, stair step or box

Lie on your back with your feet planted on top of the Bosu cross your leg. Tighten your lower abdomen, squeeze your buttocks and raise your buttocks. Brace the stomach muscles to keep your spine from moving, trying to keep the pelvis level the entire time.

_____ Reps _____ Sets _____ X Day _____ Hold		_____ Reps _____ Sets _____ X Day _____ Hold

15 | Notes: | **16** | Notes:

Starting
Position

BRIDGING CROSSED LEG - ARMS UP

Lie on your back, cross your leg and put your hands together as shown. Next, tighten your lower abdomen, squeeze your buttocks and raise your buttocks off the floor/bed. Brace the stomach muscles to keep your spine from moving, trying to keep the pelvis level the entire time.

BRIDGING CROSSED LEG - ARMS UP - BOSU - can use foam pad, stair step or box

Lie on your back with your feet planted on top of the Bosu and hands together and leg crossed. Tighten your lower abdomen, squeeze your buttocks and raise your buttocks. Brace the stomach muscles to keep your spine from moving, trying to keep the pelvis level.

		_____ Reps _____ Sets _____ X Day _____ Hold
17	**Notes:**	

Starting
Position

BRIDGE - ELASTIC BAND

Lie on your back, hold an elastic band down around your waist for resistance. Tighten your lower abdomen, squeeze your buttocks and then raise your buttocks off the floor/bed. Brace the stomach muscles to keep your spine from moving, trying to keep the pelvis level the entire time.

		_____ Reps _____ Sets _____ X Day _____ Hold
18	**Notes:**	

Starting
Position

BRIDGING - ABDUCTION - ELASTIC BAND – can be done with feet on BOSU, foam, stair step or box

Lie on your back, place an elastic band around your knees and pull your knees apart. Hold this and then tighten your lower abdomen, squeeze your buttocks and raise your buttocks off the floor/bed. Brace the stomach muscles to keep your spine from moving, trying to keep the pelvis level the entire time.

		_____ Reps _____ Sets _____ X Day _____ Hold
19	**Notes:**	

Starting
Position

FLOOR BRIDGE - EXERCISE BALL

Lie on the floor, place an exercise ball under your lower legs and then raise up your buttocks. Hold and repeat. Brace the stomach muscles to keep your spine from moving, trying to keep the pelvis level the entire time.

		_____ Reps _____ Sets _____ X Day _____ Hold
20	**Notes:**	

Starting
Position

FLOOR BRIDGE ALTERNATE LEG LIFT - EXERCISE BALL

Lie on the floor, place an exercise ball under your lower legs and then raise up your buttocks. While holding this position raise up a leg off the ball towards the ceiling then lower back to the ball and alternate to lift the other leg. Brace the stomach muscles to keep your spine from moving, trying to keep the pelvis level.

	_____ Reps _____ Sets _____ X Day _____ Hold
21	**Notes:**

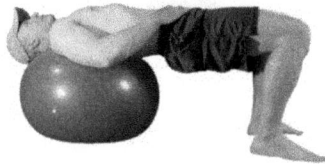

BRIDGE UPPER BACK - EXERCISE BALL

Start in a seated position on the ball and slowly walk your feet forward so that the ball is on your upper back. Keep your buttocks and pelvis up off the ball and straight with your thighs. Brace the stomach muscles to keep your spine from moving, trying to keep the pelvis level the entire time.
*To increase the challenge, you can do a supine march or perform some arm exercises, such as Fly's or Chest Presses (*See Upper Extremity exercises*)

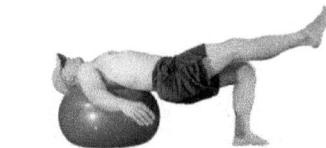

	_____ Reps _____ Sets _____ X Day _____ Hold
22	**Notes:**

Starting Position

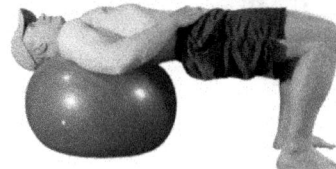

BRIDGE UPPER BACK - SINGLE LEG - EXERCISE BALL

Start in a seated position on the ball and slowly walk your feet forward so that the ball is on your upper back. Keep your buttocks and pelvis up off the ball and straight with your thighs. Raise up one leg so that you straighten your knee in the air. Return it back to the floor and then switch to raise up the other side. Brace the stomach muscles to keep your spine from moving, trying to keep the pelvis level the entire time.

Quadruped

	_____ Reps _____ Sets _____ X Day _____ Hold
23	**Notes:**

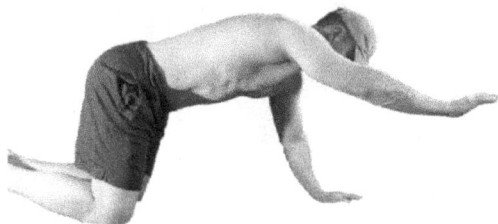

QUADRUPED ALTERNATE ARM

While in a crawling position, slowly raise up an arm out in front of you.

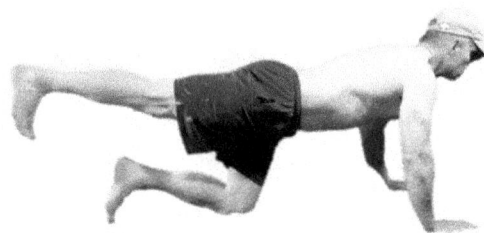

	_____ Reps _____ Sets _____ X Day _____ Hold
24	**Notes:**

QUADRUPED ALTERNATE LEG

While in a crawling position, slowly draw your leg back behind you as you straighten your knee. Either repeat on same side or alternate.

| _____ Reps _____ Sets _____X Day _____Hold |
| 25 Notes: |

QUADRUPED ALTERNATE ARM AND LEG

While in a crawling position, brace at your abdominals and then slowly lift a leg and opposite arm upwards. Maintain a level and stable pelvis and spine the entire time. Either repeat on same side or alternate.

| _____ Reps _____ Sets _____X Day _____Hold |
| 26 Notes: |

Touch your elbow to your opposite knee

Starting

Position

BIRD DOG ELBOW TOUCHES

While in a crawling position, slowly lift your leg and opposite arm upwards. When returning your arm and leg down, do not touch the floor but instead touch your elbow to your opposite knee and lift and straighten them again. Then set them down on the floor. Either repeat on same side or alternate.

| _____ Reps _____ Sets _____X Day _____Hold |
| 27 Notes: |

PRONE BALL

Lie face down over a ball, support your self with your feet and hands.

| _____ Reps _____ Sets _____X Day _____Hold |
| 28 Notes: |

PRONE BALL - ALTERNATE ARM

Lie face down over a ball, support your self with your feet and hands. Next, slowly raise up one arm. Return arm back to floor and then raise up the other arm. Keep alternating arms.

	_____ Reps _____ Sets _____X Day _____Hold		_____ Reps _____ Sets _____X Day _____Hold
29	Notes:	30	Notes:

PRONE BALL - ALTERNATE LEG

Lie face down over a ball, support yourself with your arms and legs. Next slowly raise up a leg. Return leg back to floor and then raise up the other leg.

PRONE BALL - ALTERNATE ARM AND LEG

Lie face down over a ball, support yourself with your feet and hands. Next, slowly raise up one arm and opposite leg. Return arm and leg back to floor and then raise up the opposite arm/leg.

Plank

	_____ Reps _____ Sets _____X Day _____Hold		_____ Reps _____ Sets _____X Day _____Hold
31	Notes:	32	Notes:

Starting

Position

MODIFIED PLANK

Lie face down, lift your body up on your elbows and toes. Try and maintain a straight spine the entire time. Do not allow your low back sag downward.

MODIFIED PLANK - ALTERNATE LEG

Lie face down, lift your body up on your elbows and toes. Next, lift one leg off the ground and then set it back down. Then repeat on the other leg. Try and maintain a straight spine the entire time.

_____ Reps _____ Sets _____X Day _____Hold		_____ Reps _____ Sets _____X Day _____Hold	
33	Notes:	**34**	Notes:

FULL PLANK

Lie face down, lift your body up on your elbows and toes. Straighten your arms in full elbow extension and hold in full plank position. Do not let your back arch down. Try and maintain a straight spine the entire time.

PLANK - ALTERNATE ARMS

Hold a plank position as previous (#33). Raise one arm out in front of you as shown. Return to the starting position and then raise your other arm out in front of you and repeat.
Try and maintain a straight spine the entire time.

_____ Reps _____ Sets _____X Day _____Hold		_____ Reps _____ Sets _____X Day _____Hold	
35	Notes:	**36**	Notes:

PLANK - ALTERNATE LEGS

Hold a plank position as previous (#33). Raise one leg off the floor as shown. Return to the starting position and then raise your other leg and repeat. Try and maintain a straight spine the entire time.

PLANK - EXERCISE BALL

While kneeling on the floor with an exercise ball in front of you, place your elbows and hands on the ball and lift your body up. Try and maintain a straight spine. Do not allow your hips or pelvis on either side to drop.

Back Extension

	_____ Reps _____ Sets _____X Day _____Hold		_____ Reps _____ Sets _____X Day _____Hold
37	**Notes:**	**38**	**Notes:**

PRONE ON ELBOWS

Lie face down, slowly press up and prop yourself up on your elbows.

PRESS UPS

Lie face down, slowly press up and arch your back using your arms.

	_____ Reps _____ Sets _____X Day _____Hold		_____ Reps _____ Sets _____X Day _____Hold
39	**Notes:**	**40**	**Notes:**

SKYDIVER

Lie face down with arms by your side. Next, lift your upper body, lower legs, thighs, and arms off the ground at the same time as shown. You can place a pillow under your stomach/hips for comfort.

PRONE SUPERMAN - BOSU

Lie face down over the Bosu. Slowly raise your arms and legs upward off the ground. Then lower slowly back to the ground.

_____ Reps _____ Sets _____X Day _____Hold

41 Notes:

Starting Position

TRUNK EXTENSION - BOSU

Lie face down with your upper body on a Bosu and slowly raise your head and chest upwards as shown.
Your arms can be behind your back or alongside your body.

_____ Reps _____ Sets _____X Day _____Hold

42 Notes:

Starting Position

TRUNK EXTENSION - HANDS BEHIND HEAD - BOSU

Lie face down with your upper body on a Bosu. Touch the back of your head with both hands and slowly raise your head and chest upwards.

_____ Reps _____ Sets _____X Day _____Hold

43 Notes:

Starting Position

TRUNK EXTENSION - HANDS CROSSED IN FRONT - BOSU

While lying face down with your upper body on a Bosu, slowly raise your head and chest upwards.
Keep your arms crossed on your chest as you perform.

_____ Reps _____ Sets _____X Day _____Hold

44 Notes:

SUPERMAN - ARMS BACK- EXERCISE BALL

Start in a kneeling position with an exercise ball in front of you. Roll forward so that you are face down on the ball with your feet on the ground and your stomach on the ball. Hold up your head and chest so that a straight line exists between your feet and head. Also bring your arms back along side of your body and hold this position.

	_____ Reps _____ Sets _____X Day _____Hold		_____ Reps _____ Sets _____X Day _____Hold
45	Notes:	46	Notes:

SUPERMAN – BOTH ARMS IN FRONT - EXERCISE BALL

Start in a kneeling position with an exercise ball in front of you. Next, roll forward so that you are face down on the ball with your feet on the ground and your stomach on the ball. Hold up your head and chest so that a straight line exists between your feet and head. Also bring your arms up and forward out in front of you and hold this position.

SUPERMAN – ONE ARM FORWARD / ONE ARM BACK - EXERCISE BALL

Start in a kneeling position with an exercise ball in front of you. Next, roll forward so that you are face down on the ball with your feet on the ground and your stomach on the ball. Hold up your head and chest so that a straight line exists between your feet and head. Raise one arm up and out in front of you as you bring the other arm back and along side your body as in a swimming motion.

Lateral Plank

	_____ Reps _____ Sets _____X Day _____Hold		_____ Reps _____ Sets _____X Day _____Hold
47	Notes:	48	Notes:

Starting

Position

LATERAL PLANK MODIFIED

Lie on your side with your knees bent, lift your body up on your elbow and knees. Try and maintain a straight spine.

LATERAL PLANK MODIFIED- BOSU- can be anything unstable

Lie on your side with your knees bent and your elbow on the Bosu, lift your body up on your elbow and knees. Try and maintain a straight spine.

_____ Reps _____ Sets _____X Day _____Hold

49 Notes:

LATERAL PLANK - 1 KNEE 1 FOOT

Lie on your side with bottom knee bent and top knee straight. Lift your body up on your elbow and knee on one side and foot on the other side. Try and maintain a straight spine.

_____ Reps _____ Sets _____X Day _____Hold

50 Notes:

LATERAL PLANK - 1 KNEE 1 FOOT – BOSU- Can be anything unstable

Lie on your side with elbow on Bosu with bottom knee bent and the top knee straight. Lift your body up on your elbow and knee on one side and foot on the other side. Try and maintain a straight spine.

_____ Reps _____ Sets _____X Day _____Hold

51 Notes:

Starting

Position

LATERAL PLANK

Lie on your side with both legs straight and lift your body up on your elbow and feet. Try and maintain a straight spine.

_____ Reps _____ Sets _____X Day _____Hold

52 Notes:

LATERAL PLANK - BOSU - Can be anything unstable

Lie on your side with your elbow on the Bosu and both legs straight. Lift your body up on your elbow and feet. Try and maintain a straight spine.

Backward Lean

_____ Reps _____ Sets _____ X Day _____ Hold	_____ Reps _____ Sets _____ X Day _____ Hold
53 Notes:	**54** Notes:

LEAN BACK

Start in an upright seated position with knees bent. Hold onto thighs and lean back keeping spine as straight as possible.

LEAN BACK - BOSU

Start in an upright seated position on Bosu with knees bent. Hold onto thighs or Bosu and lean back keeping spine as straight as possible.

_____ Reps _____ Sets _____ X Day _____ Hold	_____ Reps _____ Sets _____ X Day _____ Hold
55 Notes:	**56** Notes:

LEAN BACK WITH ARMS OUT

Start in an upright seated position with knees bent. Hold arms straight out or overhead, brace core and lean back keeping spine as straight as possible

LEAN BACK WITH ARMS OUT - BOSU

Start in an upright seated position on Bosu with knees bent. Hold arms straight out or overhead, brace core and lean back keeping spine as straight as possible.

_____ Reps _____ Sets _____ X Day _____ Hold		_____ Reps _____ Sets _____ X Day _____ Hold
57	Notes:	**58**	Notes:

Starting

Position

LEAN BACK WITH TWIST

Start in an upright seated position with knees bent. Hold arms straight out, brace core and lean back keeping spine as straight as possible. Rotate trunk/arms to one side and then repeat to the other side.

Starting

Position

LEAN BACK WITH TWIST – BOSU

Start in an upright seated position on Bosu with knees bent. Hold arms straight out, brace core and lean back keeping spine as straight as possible. Rotate trunk/arms to one side - repeat to the other side

_____ Reps _____ Sets _____ X Day _____ Hold		_____ Reps _____ Sets _____ X Day _____ Hold
59	Notes:	**60**	Notes:

CRUNCHY FROG

Sit on floor or edge of couch/bench. Lean back and with arms wide apart and legs straight. Next, bring knees towards chest and arms forward and return to starting position.

SEATED BIKE - FORWARD AND BACKWARDS

Sit on floor and lean back. With arms on floor or off ground, peddle feet forward for 15-30 repetitions, rest and then reverse. *Progress by moving hands forward near hips or remove arm support*

Abdominal Crunch Variations

	_____ Reps _____ Sets _____ X Day _____ Hold
61	**Notes:**

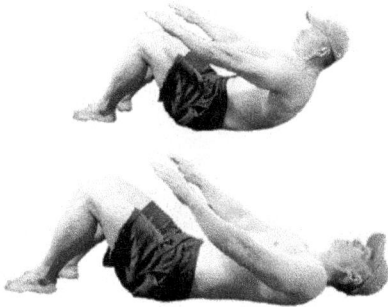

Starting Position

CRUNCH – ARMS OUT

Lie on your back with your arms outstretched forward, brace core and curl up lifting your shoulder blades off the ground. Exhale as you come up and squeeze/tighten your abdominal muscles.

	_____ Reps _____ Sets _____ X Day _____ Hold
62	**Notes:**

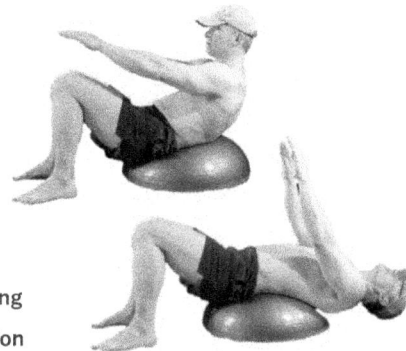

Starting Position

CRUNCH – ARMS OUT - BOSU

Lie on your back on Bosu with your arms outstretched forward, brace core and curl up lifting your shoulder blades off the ground. Exhale as you come up and squeeze/tighten your abdominal muscles.

	_____ Reps _____ Sets _____ X Day _____ Hold
63	**Notes:**

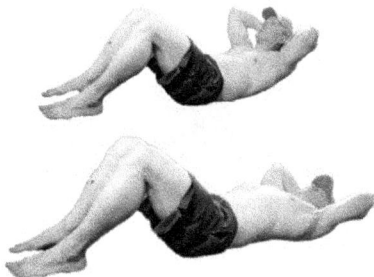

Starting Position

CRUNCH – ARMS IN BACK OF HEAD

Lie on your back with your arms behind your head, brace core and curl up lifting your shoulder blades off the ground. Exhale as you come up and squeeze/tighten your abdominal muscles. Do not pull on your neck/head.

	_____ Reps _____ Sets _____ X Day _____ Hold
64	**Notes:**

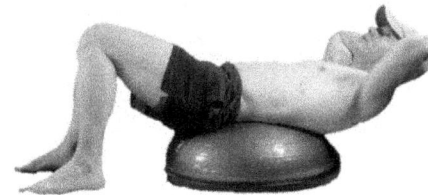

CRUNCH – ARMS IN BACK OF HEAD - BOSU

Lie on your back on Bosu with your arms behind your head, brace core and curl up lifting your shoulder blades off the ground. Exhale as you come up and squeeze/tighten your abdominal muscles. Do not pull on your neck/head.

	_____ Reps _____ Sets _____ X Day _____ Hold
65	**Notes:**

OBLIQUE CRUNCH

Lie on your back with one or both hands in back of head. Brace core and curl up targeting elbow to opposite knee as shown. Keep shoulders off floor. Exhale as you come up and squeeze/tighten your abdominal muscles. Do not pull on your neck/head.

	_____ Reps _____ Sets _____ X Day _____ Hold
66	**Notes:**

OBLIQUE CRUNCH - BOSU

Lie back on Bosu with one or both hands in back of head. Brace core and curl up targeting elbow to opposite knee as shown. Keep shoulders off Bosu. Exhale as you come up and squeeze/tighten your abdominal muscles. Do not pull on your neck/head.

	_____ Reps _____ Sets _____ X Day _____ Hold
67	**Notes:**

90 DEGREE CRUNCH

Lie on your back with legs straight in air. Reach your hands towards toes, crunching shoulders off ground. Exhale as you come up and squeeze/tighten your abdominal muscles.

	_____ Reps _____ Sets _____ X Day _____ Hold
68	**Notes:**

BALL CRUNCH – Can put legs on seat of chair

Lie on back with legs up on ball so knees and hips are at ~ 90 degrees. Cross hands over chest or behind head. Brace core and curl up lifting your shoulder blades off the ground. Exhale as you come up and squeeze/tighten your abdominal muscles. Do not pull on your neck/head.

_____ Reps _____ Sets _____X Day _____Hold

69 | Notes:

CURL UPS – ARMS ON LEGS - EXERCISE BALL

While sitting on an exercise ball, roll forward so that your back lies against the ball. Put hands on thighs/legs. Brace core and curl up lifting your shoulder blades off the ball. Exhale as you come up and squeeze/tighten your abdominal muscles.

Starting Position

_____ Reps _____ Sets _____X Day _____Hold

70 | Notes:

CURL UPS- ARMS CROSSED IN FRONT - EXERCISE BALL

While sitting on an exercise ball, roll forward so that your back lies against the ball. Cross hands over your chest. Brace core and curl up lifting your shoulder blades off the ball. Exhale as you come up and squeeze/tighten your abdominal muscles.

_____ Reps _____ Sets _____X Day _____Hold

71 | Notes:

CURL UPS – ARMS BEHIND HEAD - EXERCISE BALL

While sitting on an exercise ball, roll forward so that your back lies against the ball. Place your hands behind your head. Brace core and curl up lifting your shoulder blades off the ball. Exhale as you come up and squeeze/tighten your abdominal muscles. Do not pull on your neck/head.

_____ Reps _____ Sets _____X Day _____Hold

72 | Notes:

Starting Position

SUPINE CRUNCH TOUCH - EXERCISE BALL

Lie on the floor with your knees bend and holding a ball over your head. Bring both your knees and ball towards each other above your chest and touch your knees to the ball. Slowly return both to original positions and repeat.

____ Reps ____ Sets ____X Day ____Hold	____ Reps ____ Sets ____X Day ____Hold
73 Notes:	**74** Notes:

LOWER ABDOMINAL CRUNCH – WITH or WITHOUT BALL

Sit on a solid surface with or without a ball/pillow between your knees. Maintaining a straight spine, contract your lower abdominals. Lift both knees up. Hold and control movement back to starting position. Repeat. Can be done holding onto surface for added stability with or without ball (3rd picture)

HIGH MARCH CRUNCH

Lift knee towards chest keeping hips forward in a high march position. Continue to alternate sides while standing in place. Exhale as you come up and squeeze/tighten your abdominal muscles.

____ Reps ____ Sets ____X Day ____Hold	____ Reps ____ Sets ____X Day ____Hold
75 Notes:	**76** Notes:

Starting Position

STANDING SIDE CRUNCH

Standing with hip rotated out bring knee up towards same side elbow squeezing your obliques. Continue alternating sides while standing in place. Exhale as you come up and squeeze/tighten muscles.

Starting Position

STANDING BIKE CRUNCH

Lift knee to chest and rotate pulling opposite elbow towards knee. Continue to alternate sides while standing in place. Exhale as you come up and squeeze/tighten muscles.

Strengthening

Anaerobic - without oxygen: Single repetition with maximum resistance
Lifting lighter weights with a high number of repetitions will result in 'toning', whereas lifting heavier weights with a lower number of repetitions will result in 'bulking up'.

Benefits of strengthening	• Increases muscle fiber size and contractile strength • Increases tendon and ligament strength • Increases bone strength / bone mineral density • Improves hormonal balances-decreased cortisol • Increases Peripheral (PNS) and Central (CNS) Nervous System communication/proprioception • Improves function for ADL's (Activities of Daily Living)
Range of Motion (ROM)	Refers to the distance and direction a joint can move between the flexed position and the extended position (stretching from flexion to extension for physiological gain). It is important to be able to complete full ROM before adding resistance. ***Before strengthening (adding resistance), make sure you can go through full ROM*** unless being followed by an MD or physical/occupational therapist or other professional.
Forms of strengthening exercise	• **Isometric** – Muscles contract with no motion at the joint or change in length of the muscle. The exercises usually consist of maximal effort against an object that does not move, like a wall. • **Isotonic** – Muscles contract with motion at the joint; muscles either lengthen or shorten (*see **concentric/eccentric** below*). Tension is not constant through the range of motion. (During a bicep curl, holding a 5 lb weight, the contraction is not constant during the entire movement). Most common form of isotonic exercises use free weights with either dumbbells or a barbell. • **Concentric** – Muscle shortens, positive phase of lift. Bending the elbow in a bicep curl • **Eccentric** – Muscle lengthens, negative phase of lift or lowering. Straightening the elbow in a bicep curl. • **Isokinetic** – Muscles contract with motion at the joint; muscles either lengthen or shorten. Machines or equipment control the speed of the movement, so tension is constant providing the maximum amount of resistance throughout the entire movement.
Repetition (Reps)	Single cycle of lifting and lowering a weight in a controlled manner, moving through the form of the exercise. Example: 12 Bicep curls per set.
Set	Several repetitions performed one after another with no break between. There can be a number of reps per set and sets per exercise depending on the goal of the individual. Example: 12 reps x3 sets
Rep Maximum (RM)	The number of repetitions one can perform at a certain weight is called the Rep Maximum (RM). For example, if one could perform 10 repetitions with a 75 lbs dumbbell, then their RM for that weight would be 10RM. 1RM is the maximum weight that someone can lift in a given exercise - i.e. a weight that they can only lift once. (*Wikipedia*) (*See Bulk Up or Tone Up Below*)
Bulk up or Tone up	Do you want to 'bulk up' or 'tone up'? Although much of this depends on genetics and your ratio of slow and fast twitch fibers, discussed in the *Endurance* section, it is good to know what your goals are before starting. The average person should be able to perform at about 75% of their maximum resistance for 10 repetitions. If you can do ONE bicep curl with a 20-pound dumbbell/weight, then you should be able to do 10 with a 15 lbs. weight. (*See Set*) 20 lbs. x 75% = 15 lbs. Once you get into a routine, it will be easy for you to know when to increase the weight.

General rule of thumb	• Work from the Ground up • Order: Isometric > ROM > Eccentric > Concentric • Use assistance before resistance – Start without weight to complete range of motion and then add weight with proper form. *(See ROM above)* • Add weight: 8-12 reps x 2-3 sets of each exercise at 75% of one repetition maximum (one-rep max). • Once you reach 12 easily, you can then recheck your one-rep max. If it has increased, then increase your weight as above. • If you are looking to 'bulk up', perform low repetitions at a higher weight – up to 85-90% of the one-rep maximum. 5-8 reps x 2-3 sets. With increased weight, there is a higher risk of injury. • If you are looking to 'tone up', perform high repetitions with 65-75% of the one-rep max. 12-20 reps x 2-3 sets. • Do NOT exercise the same muscle group every day. The muscles need about 48-72 hours to repair. This includes the abdomen. **Muscle strengthening, if you are lifting weights, alternate upper and lower body with isolated abdomen exercises every other day as well. For those working out several days a week, find a schedule that works for you, but give each muscle group 48-72 hours to recover. • Cardiac/aerobic conditioning can be done daily. • Breathe!! Always exhale on the exertion. For example, when you are doing a crunch, exhale as you flexing the abs or 'curling'. Do not hold your breath. • Engage your core. Don't forget what you learned under core and balance.

Duration, Frequency, Intensity and Movement Patterns

Intensity: How *much* mental and physical *effort* it takes to sustain an activity.	This can be done using the target heart rate range THR (optimum exercise intensity levels through beats per minute, talk test or rate of perceived exertion.
Duration: How *long* the training lasts.	The higher the intensity, the shorter the duration. The American College of Sports Medicine guidelines recommend all healthy adults aged 18–65 yr should participate in moderate intensity aerobic physical activity for a minimum of 30 min on five days per week, or vigorous intensity aerobic activity for a minimum of 20 min on three days per week.
Frequency: How *often* the training occurs.	Strength training should be performed every other day or 2-3 days a week. It is important to give each muscle group 48-72 hours to recover. Alternate upper and lower body with isolated abdomen/core exercises every other day. For those working out several days a week, find a schedule that works for you as long as you give each muscle group 48 hours of recovery time.

Movement Patterns and Examples
 	
Basic movements that help to increase overall body strengthening
	• Bend and Lift: Squats, Dead Lifts and Leg presses
	   o Picking up item off floor
	• Single Leg: Step ups, Single leg stance, Lunges
	   o Walking up steps
	• Push: Shoulder press, Bench press, Push up
	   o Pushing Shopping cart or Lawn mower
	• Pull: Lat pull downs, Seated rows
	   o Vacuuming, Raking
	• Rotational
	   o Shoveling snow

EXERCISE Lower Extremity - Lying & Seated Strengthening and Range of Motion	EXERCISE NUMBER	NOTES
INVERSION – SEATED - ELASTIC BAND	1	
INVERSION – SEATED - ELASTIC BAND - 2	2	
EVERSION – SEATED - ELASTIC BAND	3	
EVERSION – SEATED - ELASTIC BAND - 2	4	
ANKLE PUMPS - SEATED	5	
ANKLE PUMPS – SUPINE or FEET UP ON STOOL	6	
DORSIFLEXION – SEATED - ELASTIC BAND	7	
DORSIFLEXION – SEATED - ELASTIC BAND - 2	8	
PLANTARFLEXION - STRAP	9	
PLANTARFLEXION - SEATED – ELASTIC BAND	10	
HEEL SLIDES - SUPINE	11	
HEEL SLIDES - RESISTED EXTENSION – ELASTIC BAND	12	
QUAD SET –ISOMETRIC	13	
QUAD SET WITH TOWEL UNDER HEEL - ISOMETRIC	14	
SHORT ARC QUAD (SAQ) – SELF ASSISTED	15	
SHORT ARC QUAD - (SAQ)	16	
KNEE EXTENSION - SELF ASSISTED	17	
PARTIAL ARC QUAD - LOW SEAT	18	
LONG ARC QUAD (LAQ) – LOW SEAT (90 deg)	19	
LONG ARC QUAD (LAQ) – LOW SEAT - ANKLE WEIGHTS	20	
LONG ARC QUAD (LAQ) - HIGH SEAT	21	
LONG ARC QUAD (LAQ) - HIGH SEAT - ANKLE WEIGHTS	22	
LONG ARC QUAD - ELASTIC BAND – HAND HELD	23	
LONG ARC QUAD - ELASTIC BAND	24	

EXERCISE Lower Extremity - Lying & Seated Strengthening and Range of Motion	EXERCISE NUMBER	NOTES
HAMSTRING CURLS - PRONE - ASSISTED	25	
HAMSTRING CURLS - PRONE	26	
HAMSTRING CURLS - - PRONE - WEIGHTS	27	
HAMSTRING CURLS – PRONE - ELASTIC BAND	28	
HAMSTRING CURLS – ELASTIC BAND	29	
HAMSTRING CURLS – ELASTIC BAND - 2	30	
HAMSTRING CURLS ON BALL	31	
HAMSTRING CURLS - SINGLE LEG - EXERCISE BALL	32	
HIP FLEXION ISOMETRIC	33	
HIP FLEXION ISOMETRIC BILATERAL	34	
HIP FLEXION – ISOMETRIC	35	
STRAIGHT LEG RAISE (SLR)	36	
STRAIGHT LEG RAISE (SLR) – ANKLE WEIGHTS	37	
STRAIGHT LEG RAISE (SLR) - ELASTIC BAND	38	
SEATED MARCHING	39	
SEATED MARCHING - ELASTIC BAND	40	
HIP EXTENSION - PRONE	41	
HIP EXTENSION – PRONE – ANKLE WEIGHTS	42	
HIP EXTENSION – PRONE – ELASTIC BAND	43	
HIP EXTENSION – QUADRUPED	44	
HIP ABDUCTION - SUPINE	45	
HIP ABDUCTION - SUPINE – ANKLE WEIGHTS	46	
HIP ABDUCTION – SUPINE - ELASTIC BAND	47	
HIP ABDUCTION / CLAMS– SUPINE - ELASTIC BAND	48	
MODIFIED HIP ABDUCTION – SIDELYING	49	

EXERCISE Lower Extremity - Lying & Seated Strengthening and Range of Motion	EXERCISE NUMBER	NOTES
HIP ABDUCTION – SIDELYING	50	
HIP ABDUCTION – SIDELYING - WEIGHTS	51	
HIP ABDUCTION – SIDELYING - ELASTIC BAND	52	
CLAM SHELLS	53	
SIDELYING CLAM - ELASTIC BAND	54	
HIP ABDUCTION - FIRE HYDRANT - QUADRUPED	55	
HIP ABDUCTION - FIRE HYDRANT – QUADRUPED - ELASTIC BAND	56	
HIP ABDUCTION - SEATED - STRAIGHT LEG	57	
HIP ABDUCTION - SEATED - STRAIGHT LEG – ANKLE WEIGHT	58	
HIP ABDUCTION - SINGLE- SEATED	59	
HIP ABDUCTION - SINGLE- SEATED – ELASTIC BAND	60	
HIP ABDUCTION - BILATERAL- SEATED	61	
HIP ABDUCTION - BILATERAL- SEATED - ELASTIC BAND	62	
HIP ADDUCTION SQUEEZE – SUPINE – KNEES BENT	63	
HIP ADDUCTION SQUEEZE – SUPINE – LEGS STRAIGHT	64	
HIP ADDUCTION - SIDELYING	65	
INTERNAL ROTATION - HEEL SQUEEZE - ISOMETRIC	67	
HIP INTERNAL ROTATION - SUPINE	68	
REVERSE CLAMS - SIDELYING	69	
REVERSE CLAMS - SIDELYING - ELASTIC BAND	70	
HIP INTERNAL ROTATION - SEATED	71	
HIP INTERNAL ROTATION - ELASTIC BAND	72	
HIP EXTERNAL ROTATION - SUPINE	73	

EXERCISE Lower Extremity - Lying & Seated Strengthening and Range of Motion	EXERCISE NUMBER	NOTES
HIP EXTERNAL ROTATION - ELASTIC BAND	74	
HIP ROTATIONS – BILATERAL - SIDELYING	75	
HIP ROTATION - SEATED - BALL and ELASTIC BAND	76	
PRESS – BILATERAL – ELASTIC BAND	77	
PRESS – SINGLE LEG – ELASTIC BAND	78	
HIP HIKE - STANDING	79	
HIP HIKE – KNEELING	80	
GLUTE SETS - PRONE	81	
GLUTE SET - SUPINE	82	
GLUTE SQUEEZE - SITTING	83	
PT (MAX/MEDIUS)	84	

LOWER EXTREMITY - Range Of Motion > Isometric > Strength
Lying and Seated

Inversion (IV) / Eversion (EV)

	_____ Reps _____ Sets _____ X Day _____ Hold
1	**Notes:**

INVERSION – SEATED - ELASTIC BAND

In a seated position, cross your legs and using an elastic band attached to your foot, hook it under your opposite foot and up to your hand. Draw the resisted foot inward. Keep your heel in contact with the floor the entire time.

	_____ Reps _____ Sets _____ X Day _____ Hold
2	**Notes:**

INVERSION – SEATED - ELASTIC BAND - 2

In a seated position, use an elastic band secured to a steady object and the other end attached to your foot. Draw the resisted foot inward. Keep your heel in contact with the floor the entire time.

	_____ Reps _____ Sets _____ X Day _____ Hold
3	**Notes:**

EVERSION – SEATED - ELASTIC BAND

In a seated position, use an elastic band attached to your foot, hook it under your opposite foot and up to your hand. Draw the resisted foot outward. Keep your heel in contact with the floor the entire time.

	_____ Reps _____ Sets _____ X Day _____ Hold
4	**Notes:**

EVERSION – SEATED - ELASTIC BAND - 2

In a seated position, use an elastic band secured to a steady object and the other end attached to your foot. Draw the resisted foot outward. Keep your heel in contact with the floor the entire time.

Dorsiflexion (DF) / Plantarflexion (PF)

	_____ Reps _____ Sets _____ X Day _____ Hold
5	**Notes:**

ANKLE PUMPS - SEATED

In a seated position keeping feet on the floor, first go up on toes (toes pointed towards the ground – PF). Then point toes up keeping heels on the ground (DF). Alternate back and forth in a pumping motion.

	_____ Reps _____ Sets _____ X Day _____ Hold
6	**Notes:**

ANKLE PUMPS – SUPINE or FEET UP ON STOOL

Lying or with feet up on stool first point the toes forward (PF) and then back up with toes facing the ceiling. Alternate back and forth in a pumping motion.

	_____ Reps _____ Sets _____ X Day _____ Hold
7	**Notes:**

DORSIFLEXION – SEATED - ELASTIC BAND

In a seated position, use an elastic band attached to your target foot, hook it under your opposite foot and up to your hand. Draw the band upwards with the resisted foot as shown. Keep your heel in contact with the floor the entire time.

	_____ Reps _____ Sets _____ X Day _____ Hold
8	**Notes:**

DORSIFLEXION – SEATED - ELASTIC BAND - 2

In a seated position, use an elastic band secured to a steady object and the other end attached to your foot. Draw the resisted foot upward. Keep your heel in contact with the floor the entire time.

	_____ Reps _____ Sets _____X Day _____Hold			_____ Reps _____ Sets _____X Day _____Hold
9	Notes:		10	Notes:

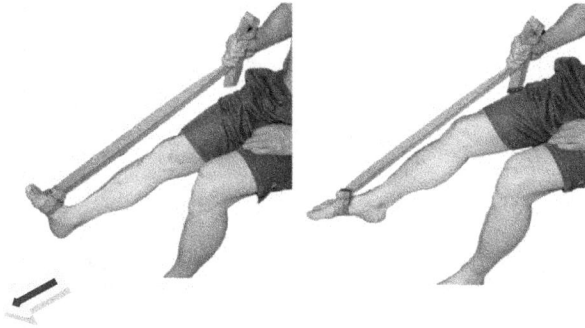

PLANTARFLEXION - STRAP

In a seated position, attach one loop of the strap to your foot and hold the other end. Move your foot forward and back at the ankle as shown. Keep your heel in contact with the floor the entire time.

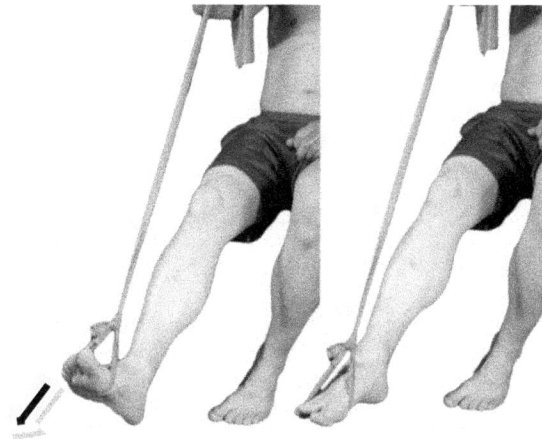

PLANTARFLEXION - SEATED – ELASTIC BAND

In a seated position, hold an elastic band and attach the other end to your foot. Press your foot downward towards the floor. Keep your heel in contact with the floor the entire time.

Heel Slides

	_____ Reps _____ Sets _____X Day _____Hold			_____ Reps _____ Sets _____X Day _____Hold
11	Notes:		12	Notes:

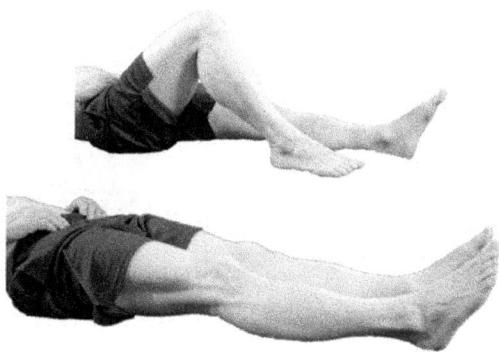

HEEL SLIDES - SUPINE

Lie on your back with knees straight and slide the target heel towards your buttock as you bend your knee. Hold a gentle stretch in this position and then return to original position.

Starting Position

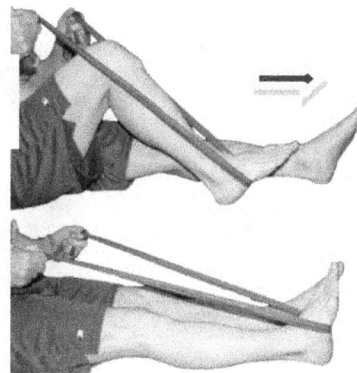

HEEL SLIDES - RESISTED EXTENSION – ELASTIC BAND

Long sit with band around bottom of target foot. Slide the target heel towards your buttock as you bend your knee. Push your foot to straighten knee against resistance to the original position.

Quadriceps (QUAD) / Knee Extension

	_____ Reps _____ Sets _____ X Day _____ Hold		_____ Reps _____ Sets _____ X Day _____ Hold
13	Notes:	**14**	Notes:

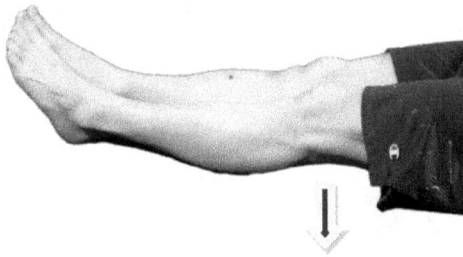

QUAD SET –ISOMETRIC

Tighten your top thigh muscle as you attempt to press the back of your knee downward towards the table. Hold 5-10 seconds. Repeat.

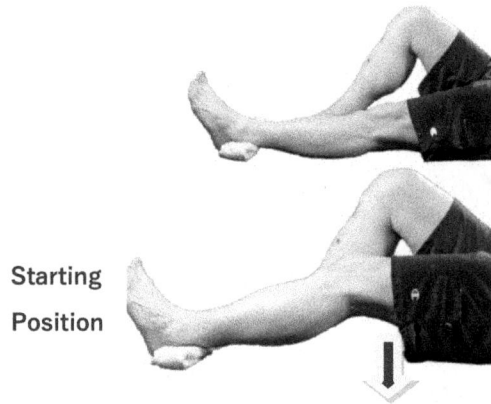

Starting Position

QUAD SET WITH TOWEL UNDER HEEL - ISOMETRIC

Lying or sitting with a small towel roll under your ankle, tighten your top thigh muscle to press the back of your knee downward towards the ground. Hold 5-10 seconds. Repeat.

	_____ Reps _____ Sets _____ X Day _____ Hold		_____ Reps _____ Sets _____ X Day _____ Hold
15	Notes:	**16**	Notes:

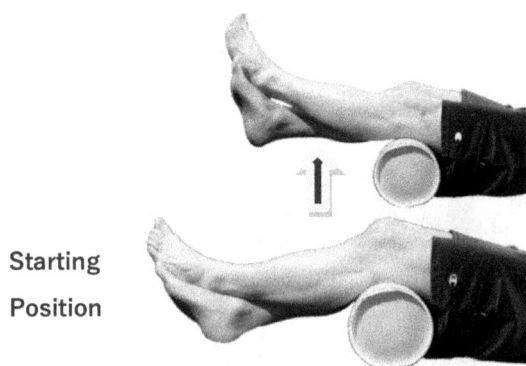

Starting Position

SHORT ARC QUAD (SAQ) – SELF ASSISTED

Place a rolled-up towel or other rounded object under your knee. Hook one foot under the other to assist the affected leg. Slowly straighten your knee as your raise up your foot tightening the top thigh muscle.

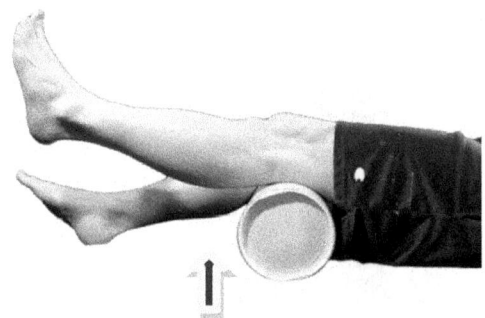

SHORT ARC QUAD - (SAQ) - Can add ankle weight

Place a rolled-up towel or object under your knee and slowly straighten your knee as your raise up your foot tightening the top thigh muscle. Flex your foot to increase the stretch.

	_____ Reps _____ Sets _____X Day _____Hold
17	**Notes:**

KNEE EXTENSION - SELF ASSISTED

In a seated position, place the unaffected leg under the target leg. Use the unaffected leg to assist the target leg up to a straightened knee position.

	_____ Reps _____ Sets _____X Day _____Hold
18	**Notes:**

PARTIAL ARC QUAD - LOW SEAT - Can add ankle weight

Sit with your knee in a semi bent position and your heel touching the ground and then slowly straighten your knee as you raise your foot upwards as shown. Lower your foot back down slowly controling the muscle until your heel touches the ground and then repeat.

	_____ Reps _____ Sets _____X Day _____Hold
19	**Notes:**

LONG ARC QUAD (LAQ) – LOW SEAT (90 deg)

Sit with your knee in a bent position and then tighten the quadricep. Slowly straighten your knee as you raise your foot upwards as shown. Lower your foot back down to original bent knee position slowly controlling the muscle and then repeat.

	_____ Reps _____ Sets _____X Day _____Hold
20	**Notes:**

LONG ARC QUAD (LAQ) – LOW SEAT - ANKLE WEIGHTS

Attach and ankle weight. Sit with your knee in a bent position and then tighten the quadricep. Slowly straighten your knee as you raise your foot upwards as shown. Lower your foot back down to original bent knee position slowly controlling the muscle - repeat.

	_____ Reps _____ Sets _____ X Day _____ Hold
21	Notes:

LONG ARC QUAD (LAQ) - HIGH SEAT

Sit with your knee in a bent position and then tighten the quadricep. Slowly straighten your knee as you raise your foot upwards as shown. Lower your foot back down to original bent knee position slowly controlling the muscle and then repeat.

	_____ Reps _____ Sets _____ X Day _____ Hold
22	Notes:

LONG ARC QUAD (LAQ) - HIGH SEAT - ANKLE WEIGHTS

Attach and ankle weight. Sit with your knee in a bent position and then tighten the quadricep. Slowly straighten your knee as you raise your foot upwards as shown. Lower your foot back down to original bent knee position slowly controlling the muscle and then repeat.

	_____ Reps _____ Sets _____ X Day _____ Hold
23	Notes:

LONG ARC QUAD - ELASTIC BAND – HANDHELD

Attach a looped elastic band to your ankle and to the opposite foot or hold with your hand. Sit with your knee in a bent position and then tighten the quadricep. Draw your lower leg upwards to a straighten knee position while your other foot or hand secures the band. Lower your foot back down to original bent knee position slowly controlling the muscle and then repeat.

	_____ Reps _____ Sets _____ X Day _____ Hold
24	Notes:

LONG ARC QUAD - ELASTIC BAND

Attach a looped elastic band to your ankle and to a steady object behind you. Sit with your knee in a bent position and then tighten the quadricep. Draw your lower leg upwards to a straightened knee position. Lower your foot back down to original bent knee position slowly controlling the muscle and then repeat.

Hamstrings

	_____ Reps _____ Sets _____ X Day _____ Hold

25 | Notes:

HAMSTRING CURLS - PRONE - ASSISTED

Lie face down and hook one foot under the other to assist the affected leg. Bend the target leg with the assistance of your unaffected leg.

	_____ Reps _____ Sets _____ X Day _____ Hold

26 | Notes:

HAMSTRING CURLS - PRONE

Lie face down and slowly bend your knee as you bring your foot towards your buttock.

	_____ Reps _____ Sets _____ X Day _____ Hold

27 | Notes:

HAMSTRING CURLS - - PRONE - WEIGHTS

Attach and ankle weight. Lie face down and slowly bend your knee as you bring your foot towards your buttock.

	_____ Reps _____ Sets _____ X Day _____ Hold

28 | Notes:

HAMSTRING CURLS – PRONE - ELASTIC BAND

Attach an elastic band around your foot and opposite ankle as shown. While lying face down, slowly bend your target knee as you bring your foot towards your buttock. Keep your other foot on the floor to fixate the band.

_____ Reps _____ Sets _____X Day _____Hold		_____ Reps _____ Sets _____X Day _____Hold	
29	Notes:	**30**	Notes:

HAMSTRING CURLS – ELASTIC BAND

Sit and use an elastic band secured to a steady object and the other end attached to your ankle. Bend your knee and draw back your foot.

HAMSTRING CURLS – ELASTIC BAND - 2

Attach a looped elastic band to your ankle and to the opposite foot while one leg is propped on stool or another raised object. Draw your lower leg downwards to a bent knee position while your other ankle anchors the band on the chair.

_____ Reps _____ Sets _____X Day _____Hold		_____ Reps _____ Sets _____X Day _____Hold	
31	Notes:	**32**	Notes: **Advanced**

HAMSTRING CURLS ON BALL – can add ankle weight.

Lie prone on an exercise ball as shown. Slowly bend your knee as you bring your foot towards your buttock.

Starting

Position

HAMSTRING CURLS - SINGLE LEG - EXERCISE BALL

Lie on the floor and place your heel on an exercise ball.
Lift your buttocks and then bend your knees to draw the ball towards your buttocks. Keep your buttocks elevated off the floor the entire time.

Hip Flexion

	_____ Reps _____ Sets _____ X Day _____ Hold
33	**Notes:**

HIP FLEXION ISOMETRIC

Lie on your back, lift up your knee and press it into your hand. Hold. Return to the original position and repeat.

HIP FLEXION ISOMETRIC - ALTERNATING
Lie on your back, lift up your knee and press it into your hand. Hold. Return to the original position and repeat on the other side.

	_____ Reps _____ Sets _____ X Day _____ Hold
34	**Notes:**

HIP FLEXION ISOMETRIC BILATERAL

Lie on your back, lift up your knees and press them into your hands. Hold. Return to the original position and repeat.

	_____ Reps _____ Sets _____ X Day _____ Hold
35	**Notes:**

HIP FLEXION – ISOMETRIC - Can use towel roll for comfort

While standing in front of a wall, draw your knee forward and press it into the wall. Place a folded towel between your knee and the wall for comfort if needed.

	_____ Reps _____ Sets _____ X Day _____ Hold
36	**Notes:**

STRAIGHT LEG RAISE (SLR)

Lie on your back, tighten the quad of the target leg and lift up with a straight knee. Keep the opposite knee bent with the foot planted on the ground. (see #37 for starting position)

	_____ Reps _____ Sets _____X Day _____Hold
37	Notes:

STRAIGHT LEG RAISE (SLR) – ANKLE WEIGHTS

Attach ankle weights. Lie on your back and lift up your leg with a straight knee. Keep the opposite knee bent with the foot planted on the ground

	_____ Reps _____ Sets _____X Day _____Hold
38	Notes:

STRAIGHT LEG RAISE (SLR) - ELASTIC BAND

Lie on your back with an elastic band looped around your ankles, lift the target leg upwards.

	_____ Reps _____ Sets _____X Day _____Hold
39	Notes:

SEATED MARCHING - can add ankle weights for resistance

Sit in a chair and move a knee upward, set it back down and then alternate to the other side

	_____ Reps _____ Sets _____X Day _____Hold
40	Notes:

SEATED MARCHING - ELASTIC BAND

Sit in a chair with an elastic band wrapped around your thighs. Move a knee upward, set it back down and then alternate to the other side.

Hip Extension

_____ Reps _____ Sets _____ X Day _____ Hold	_____ Reps _____ Sets _____ X Day _____ Hold
41 Notes:	**42** Notes:

HIP EXTENSION - PRONE

Lie face down with your knee straight and slowly lift up leg off the ground. Maintain a straight knee the entire time.

HIP EXTENSION – PRONE – ANKLE WEIGHTS

Attach ankle weights. Lie face down with your knee straight and slowly lift up leg off the ground. Maintain a straight knee the entire time.

_____ Reps _____ Sets _____ X Day _____ Hold	_____ Reps _____ Sets _____ X Day _____ Hold
43 Notes:	**44** Notes:

HIP EXTENSION – PRONE – ELASTIC BAND

Lie on your stomach with an elastic band looped around your ankles and lift the targeted leg upwards. Maintain a straight knee the entire time.

HIP EXTENSION – QUADRUPED with or without ankle weights

Start in a crawl position and then raise your leg up behind you as shown. Keep your knee bent at 90 degrees the entire time.

Hip Abduction (ABD)

	_____ Reps _____ Sets _____X Day _____Hold		_____ Reps _____ Sets _____X Day _____Hold
45	**Notes:**	**46**	**Notes:**

HIP ABDUCTION - SUPINE

Lie on your back and slowly bring your leg out to the side. Return to original position and repeat. Keep your knee straight the entire time.

HIP ABDUCTION - SUPINE – ANKLE WEIGHTS

Attach and weights. Lie on your back and slowly bring your leg up slightly and then out to the side. Return to original position and repeat. Keep your knee straight the entire time.

	_____ Reps _____ Sets _____X Day _____Hold		_____ Reps _____ Sets _____X Day _____Hold
47	**Notes:**	**48**	**Notes:**

HIP ABDUCTION – SUPINE - ELASTIC BAND

Lie on your back and slowly bring your leg out to the side. Return to original position and repeat. Keep your knee straight the entire time.

HIP ABDUCTION / CLAMS– SUPINE - ELASTIC BAND

Lie down on your back with your knees bent. Place an elastic band around your knees and then draw your knees apart. Return to original position and repeat.

	_____ Reps _____ Sets _____X Day _____Hold
49	**Notes:**

MODIFIED HIP ABDUCTION – SIDELYING can add weights

Lie on your side and slowly lift up your top leg to the side. The bottom leg can be bent to stabilize your body. Keep your knee straight and maintain your toes pointed forward the entire time. Keep your leg in-line with your body. Return to original position and repeat.

	_____ Reps _____ Sets _____X Day _____Hold
50	**Notes:**

HIP ABDUCTION – SIDELYING

Lie on your side and slowly lift up your top leg to the side. Keep your knee straight and maintain your toes pointed forward the entire time. Keep your leg in-line with your body. Return to original position and repeat.

	_____ Reps _____ Sets _____X Day _____Hold
51	**Notes:**

HIP ABDUCTION – SIDELYING - WEIGHTS

Attach ankle weights. Lie on your side and slowly lift up your top leg to the side. Keep your knee straight and maintain your toes pointed forward the entire time. Keep your leg in-line with your body. Return to original position and repeat.

	_____ Reps _____ Sets _____X Day _____Hold
52	**Notes:**

HIP ABDUCTION – SIDELYING - ELASTIC BAND

Lie on your side with an elastic band looped around your ankles. Lift the top leg upwards keeping your knee straight and maintaining your toes pointed forward the entire time. Keep your leg in-line with your body. Return to original position and repeat.

	_____ Reps _____ Sets _____X Day _____Hold
53	Notes:

Starting
Position

CLAM SHELLS

Lie on your side with your knees bent, draw up the top knee while keeping contact of your feet together.
Do not let your pelvis roll back during the lifting movement.

	_____ Reps _____ Sets _____X Day _____Hold
54	Notes:

Starting
Position

SIDELYING CLAM - ELASTIC BAND

Lie on your side with your knees bent and an elastic band wrapped around your knees, draw up the top knee while keeping contact of your feet together as shown. Do not let your pelvis roll back during the lifting movement.

	_____ Reps _____ Sets _____X Day _____Hold
55	Notes:

Starting
Position

HIP ABDUCTION - FIRE HYDRANT - QUADRUPED

Start in a crawl position and raise your leg out to the side as shown. Maintain a straight upper and mid back.

	_____ Reps _____ Sets _____X Day _____Hold
56	Notes:

Starting
Position

HIP ABDUCTION - FIRE HYDRANT – QUADRUPED - ELASTIC BAND

Start in a crawl position with an elastic band around your thighs. Raise your leg out to the side as shown. Maintain a straight upper and mid back.

	_____ Reps _____ Sets _____ X Day _____ Hold
57	**Notes:**

HIP ABDUCTION - SEATED - STRAIGHT LEG

Sit close to the edge of a chair with your target leg straight at the knee. Move your target leg to the side lifting slightly off the ground and then return to straight ahead.. You can slide your heel across the floor as you move and then return to straight ahead if unable to lift. Maintain your toes pointed up the entire time.

	_____ Reps _____ Sets _____ X Day _____ Hold
58	**Notes:**

HIP ABDUCTION - SEATED - STRAIGHT LEG – ANKLE WEIGHT

Attach an ankle weight. Sit close to the edge of a chair with your target leg straight at the knee. Move your target leg to the side lifting slightly off the ground and then return to straight ahead. Maintain your toes pointed up the entire time.

	_____ Reps _____ Sets _____ X Day _____ Hold
59	**Notes:**

HIP ABDUCTION - SINGLE- SEATED

Sit close to the edge of a chair with knees bent and both feet on the floor. Move your target knee out to the side as shown and then return to straight ahead. Maintain contact of your feet on the floor the entire time.

	_____ Reps _____ Sets _____ X Day _____ Hold
60	**Notes:**

HIP ABDUCTION - SINGLE- SEATED – ELASTIC BAND

With band tied around the thighs, sit close to the edge of a chair with knees bent and both feet on the floor. Move your target knee out to the side as shown and then return to straight ahead. Maintain contact of your feet on the floor the entire time.tact of your feet on the floor the entire time.

	_____ Reps _____ Sets _____X Day _____Hold		_____ Reps _____ Sets _____X Day _____Hold
61	Notes:	**62**	Notes:

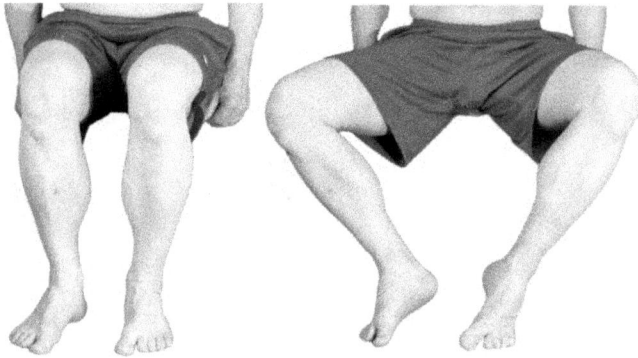

HIP ABDUCTION - BILATERAL- SEATED

Sit close to the edge of a chair with knees bent and both feet on the floor. Move your knees out to the side as shown and then return to straight ahead. Maintain contact of your feet on the floor the entire time.

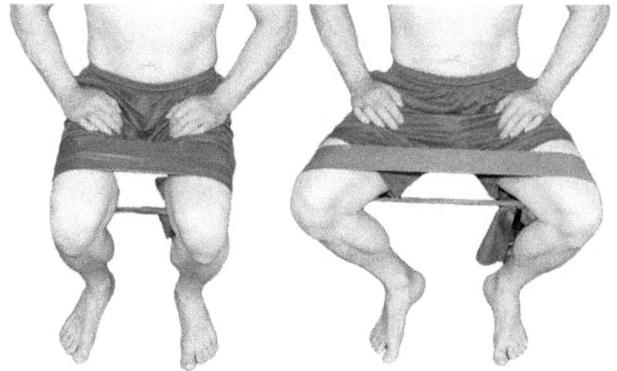

HIP ABDUCTION - BILATERAL- SEATED - ELASTIC BAND

Sit close to the edge of a chair with an elastic band wrapped around your knees. Move both knees to the sides to separate your legs. Keep contact of your feet on the floor the entire time.

Hip Adduction (ADD)

	_____ Reps _____ Sets _____X Day _____Hold		_____ Reps _____ Sets _____X Day _____Hold
63	Notes:	**64**	Notes:

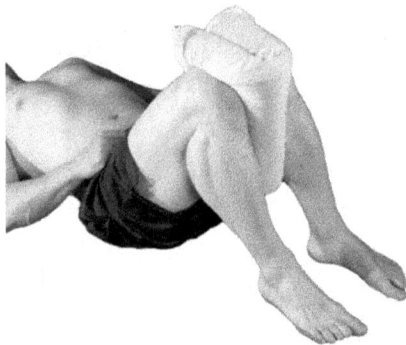

HIP ADDUCTION SQUEEZE – SUPINE – KNEES BENT

Lie on your back with legs bent and place a rolled up towel, ball or pillow between your knees. Press your knees together so that you squeeze the object firmly. Hold, release and repeat.

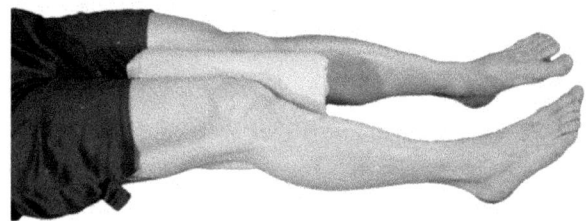

HIP ADDUCTION SQUEEZE – SUPINE – LEGS STRAIGHT

Lie on your back and place a rolled up towel, ball or pillow between your knees. Squeeze the object with your knees. Hold, release and repeat.

_____ Reps _____ Sets _____ X Day _____ Hold	_____ Reps _____ Sets _____ X Day _____ Hold
65 Notes:	**66** Notes:

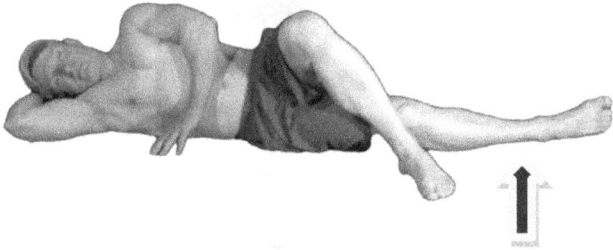

HIP ADDUCTION - SIDELYING

Lie on your side, slowly lift up your bottom leg towards the ceiling. Keep your knee straight the entire time. Your top leg should be bent at the knee and your foot planted on the ground supporting your body.

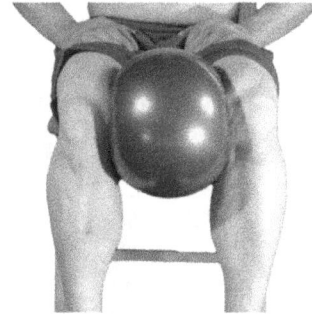

BALL SQUEEZE - SEATED

Sit and place a rolled-up towel, ball or pillow between your knees and squeeze the object firmly. Hold, release and repeat.

Hip Internal Rotation (IR)

_____ Reps _____ Sets _____ X Day _____ Hold	_____ Reps _____ Sets _____ X Day _____ Hold
67 Notes:	**68** Notes:

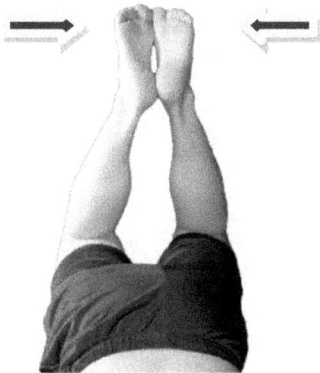

INTERNAL ROTATION - HEEL SQUEEZE - ISOMETRIC

Lie face down, spead your knees apart and press your heels together. Hold, release and repeat.

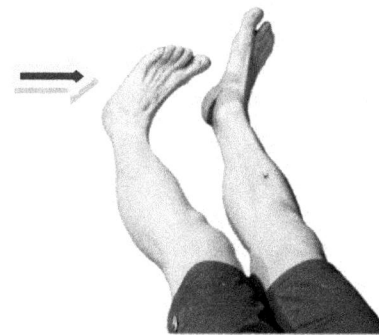

HIP INTERNAL ROTATION - SUPINE

Lie on your back with your knees straight, roll your hip in so that your toes point inward. Be sure that your knee cap faces inward as well.

_____ Reps _____ Sets _____ X Day _____ Hold

69 | Notes:

Starting
Position

REVERSE CLAMS - SIDELYING

Lie on your side with your knees bent and raise your top foot towards the ceiling while keeping contact of your knees together. Lower back down to original position. Do not let your pelvis roll forward during the lifting movement.

_____ Reps _____ Sets _____ X Day _____ Hold

70 | Notes:

Starting Position

REVERSE CLAMS - SIDELYING - ELASTIC BAND

Lie on your side with your knees bent and an elastic band around your ankles. Raise your top foot towards the ceiling while keeping contact of your knees together. Lower back down to original position. Do not let your pelvis roll forward during the lifting movement.

_____ Reps _____ Sets _____ X Day _____ Hold

71 | Notes:

HIP INTERNAL ROTATION - SEATED

Sit on a chair with your legs spread apart and feet planted on the ground. Use your hand on the inside of your knee to resist the movement inward.

_____ Reps _____ Sets _____ X Day _____ Hold

72 | Notes:

HIP INTERNAL ROTATION - ELASTIC BAND - High chair

Attach one end of an elastic band at your ankle and the other to a sturdy object. Pull away from your other leg while keeping your thigh from moving.

Hip External Rotation (ER)

_____ Reps	_____ Sets	_____ X Day	_____ Hold		

73 | Notes:

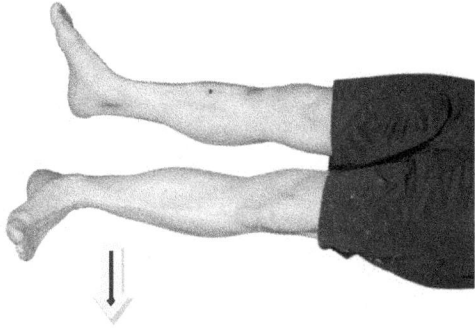

HIP EXTERNAL ROTATION - SUPINE

Lie on your back with your knees straight and roll your hip out so that your toes point outward. Be sure that your knee cap faces outward as well.

_____ Reps	_____ Sets	_____ X Day	_____ Hold

74 | Notes:

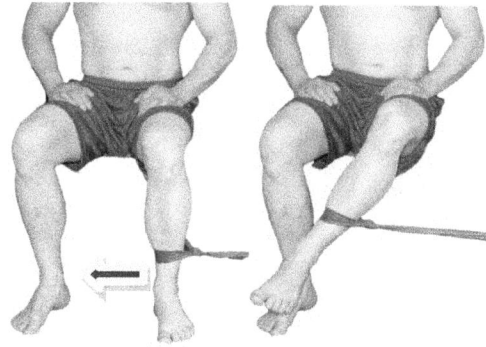

HIP EXTERNAL ROTATION - ELASTIC BAND

Sit and use an elastic band secured to a steady object and the other end attached to your ankle from the side.
Pull towards your other leg while keeping your thigh from moving across the table.

Bilateral Hip Rotation

_____ Reps	_____ Sets	_____ X Day	_____ Hold

75 | Notes:

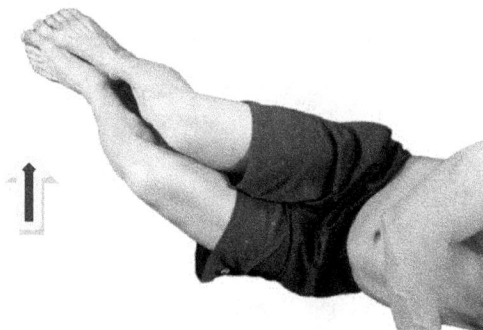

HIP ROTATIONS – BILATERAL - SIDELYING

Lie on your side in fetal position with knees and hips bent.
Slowly raise up both lower legs and feet as shown.
Your feet and knees should be touching the entire time.

_____ Reps	_____ Sets	_____ X Day	_____ Hold

76 | Notes:

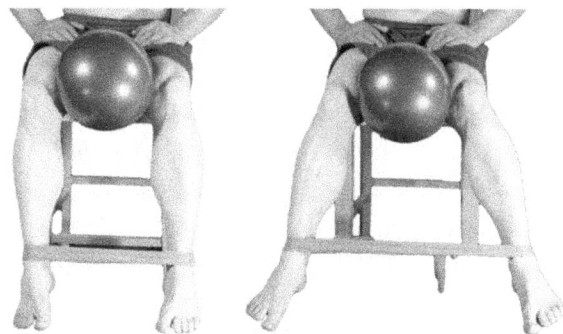

HIP ROTATION - SEATED - BALL and ELASTIC BAND – High chair

Sit and place a rolled-up towel, ball or pillow between your knees and an elastic band around your ankles. Squeeze the ball, sustain and hold. Next, pull the band as you move your feet apart from each other.

Leg Press

	_____ Reps _____ Sets _____X Day _____Hold		_____ Reps _____ Sets _____X Day _____Hold
77	Notes:	78	Notes:

Starting
Position

PRESS – BILATERAL – ELASTIC BAND

Lie on back put elastic band on bottom of both feet. Start with knees bent and push with feet to straighten both legs.

PRESS – SINGLE LEG – ELASTIC BAND

Lie on back put elastic band on bottom of one foot. Start with knees bent and push with foot to straighten leg.

Hip Hikes (Gluteus Medius)

	_____ Reps _____ Sets _____X Day _____Hold		_____ Reps _____ Sets _____X Day _____Hold
79	Notes:	80	Notes:

HIP HIKE - STANDING on Step or Pad

Stand with one foot on a step or pad and the other hanging off as shown. Raise and lower the side of your pelvis that is hanging off the edge.

HIP HIKE – KNEELING on towel or pad

Kneel on both knees with one knee on a folded towel or pad. Raise and lower the side of your pelvis that is not on the towel/pad.

Glutes (Glute Max)

_____ Reps _____ Sets _____X Day _____Hold	_____ Reps _____ Sets _____X Day _____Hold
81 Notes:	**82** Notes:

GLUTE SETS - PRONE

Lie face down, squeeze your buttocks and hold. Repeat.

GLUTE SET - SUPINE

Lie on your back, squeeze your buttocks and hold. Repeat.

_____ Reps _____ Sets _____X Day _____Hold	_____ Reps _____ Sets _____X Day _____Hold
83 Notes:	**84** Notes:

GLUTE SQUEEZE - SITTING

While sitting, squeeze your buttocks and hold. Repeat.

GLUTE SCULPT (MAX/MEDIUS)

Lie on your side leaning towards your stomach. Bend leg on target side, raise up and hold.

EXERCISE Upper Extremity Strengthening and Range of Motion	EXERCISE NUMBER	NOTES
ELBOW FLEXION EXTENSION - SUPINE	1	
ELBOW FLEXION / EXTENSION - GRAVITY ELIMINATED	2	
BICEPS CURLS – ALTERNATING	3	
BICEPS CURL - SELF FIXATION – ELASTIC BAND	4	
SEATED BICEPS CURLS - ALTERNATING	5	
SEATED BICEPS CURLS - BILATERAL	6	
CONCENTRATION CURLS – SITTING	7	
PREACHER CURL ON BALL	8	
BICEPS CURLS	9	
BICEPS CURLS - RADIOBRACHIALIS - HAMMER CURL	10	
BICEPS CURLS - BRACHIALIS	11	
BICEPS CURLS – ROTATE OUTWARD	12	
BICEPS CURLS – ONE ARM - ELASTIC BAND	13	
BICEPS CURLS – BILATERAL - ELASTIC BAND	14	
BICEPS CURLS - RADIOBRACHIALIS - HAMMER CURL – ONE ARM - ELASTIC BAND	15	
BICEPS CURLS - RADIOBRACHIALIS - HAMMER CURL – BILATERAL - ELASTIC BAND	16	
BICEPS CURLS – BRACHIALIS - ONE ARM - ELASTIC BAND	17	
BICEPS CURL – BRACHIALIS – BILATERAL - ELASTIC BAND	18	
TRICEPS - SELF FIXATION - ELASTIC BAND	19	
OVERHEAD TRICEPS - SELF FIXATION –SEATED OR STANDING - ELASTIC BAND	20	
TRICEP EXTENSION – SITTING OR STANDING - WEIGHT	21	
TRICEP EXTENSION – SITTING OR STANDING – BILATERAL - WEIGHT	22	
ELBOW EXTENSION - BALL	23	

EXERCISE Upper Extremity Strengthening and Range of Motion	EXERCISE NUMBER	NOTES
ELBOW EXTENSION - SKULL CRUSHER - BALL	24	
TRICEPS - ELASTIC BAND	25	
TRICEPS - BENT OVER	26	
CHAIR DIPS / PUSH UPS	27	
DIPS OFF CHAIR	28	
PENDULUM SHOULDER FORWARD/BACK	29	
PENDULUM SHOULDER – SIDE TO SIDE	30	
PENDULUM SHOULDER CIRCLES	31	
PENDULUMS - SUPINE	32	
ISOMETRIC FLEXION	33	
SHOULDER FLEXION – SIDELYING	34	
FLEXION – SUPINE - SINGLE OR BILATERAL	35	
FLEXION – SUPINE – SINGLE OR BILATERAL - WEIGHT	36	
FLEXION – SUPINE - DOWEL	37	
FLEXION – SUPINE - DOWEL - Weight	38	
FLEXION - SELF FIXATION – ELASTIC BAND	39	
FLEXION – ELASTIC BAND	40	
FLEXION - STANDING - PALMS DOWN / OVERHAND DOWEL	41	
FLEXION - STANDING - PALMS UP / UNDERHAND DOWEL	42	
FLEXION – PALMS FACING INWARD	43	
FLEXION – PALMS DOWN	44	
V RAISE	45	
V RAISE – WEIGHTS	46	
MILITARY PRESS – DOWEL	47	
MILITARY PRESS - FREE WEIGHTS	48	

EXERCISE Upper Extremity Strengthening and Range of Motion	EXERCISE NUMBER	NOTES
ISOMETRIC EXTENSION	49	
PRONE EXTENSION - EXERCISE BALL	50	
SHOULDER EXTENSION - STANDING	51	
SHOULDER EXTENSION - STANDING - WEIGHTS	52	
EXTENSION – STANDING – DOWEL	53	
EXTENSION - SELF FIXATION - ELASTIC BAND	54	
EXTENSION - ELASTIC BAND	55	
EXTENSION - BILATERAL - ELASTIC BAND	56	
INTERNAL ROTATION – ISOMETRIC	57	
INTERNAL ROTATION - ISOMETRIC- ELEVATED	58	
INTERNAL ROTATION - SIDELYING	59	
INTERNAL ROTATION - ELASTIC BAND	60	
INTERNAL / EXTERNAL ROTATION - STANDING – DOWEL	61	
INTERNAL ROTATION – DOWEL	62	
EXTERNAL ROTATION - ISOMETRIC	63	
EXTERNAL ROTATION - ISOMETRIC – ELEVATED	64	
EXTERNAL ROTATION WITH TOWEL - SIDELYING	65	
EXTERNAL ROTATION – 90/90 - WEIGHTS	66	
EXTERNAL ROTATION - BILATERAL - ELASTIC BAND	67	
EXTERNAL ROTATION - ELASTIC BAND	68	
ADDUCTION – ISOMETRIC	69	
ADDUCTION - ELASTIC BAND	70	
ABDUCTION – ISOMETRIC	71	
HORIZONTAL ABDUCTION - DOWEL	72	

EXERCISE Upper Extremity Strengthening and Range of Motion	EXERCISE NUMBER	NOTES
HORIZONTAL ABDUCTION/ADDUCTTION - SUPINE	73	
HORIZONTAL ABDUCTION/ADDUCTTION - SUPINE -WEIGHT	74	
ABDUCTION - SIDELYING	75	
HORIZONTAL ABDUCTION - SIDELYING	76	
ABDUCTION – WEIGHT	77	
ABDUCTION – ELASTIC BAND	78	
HORIZONTAL ABDUCTION – BILATERAL - ELASTIC BAND	79	
90/90 ABDUCTION - WEIGHT	80	
LATERAL RAISES	81	
LATERAL RAISES – LEAN FORWARD	82	
LATERAL RAISES – LEAN FORWARD - ARM ROTATION	83	
FRONTAL RAISE – WEIGHTS	84	
UPRIGHT ROW – WEIGHTS	85	
UPRIGHT ROW – ELASTIC BAND	86	
SHRUGS	87	
SHRUGS - WEIGHTS	88	
SHOULDER ROLLS	89	
SHOULDER ROLLS - WEIGHTS	90	
SCAPULAR RETRACTIONS - BILATERAL	91	
SCAPULAR RETRACTION – SINGLE ARM	92	
ELASTIC BAND SCAPULAR RETRACTIONS WITH MINI SHOULDER EXTENSIONS	93	
PRONE RETRACTION	94	
SCAPULAR PROTRACTION - SUPINE - BILATERAL	95	
SCAPULAR PROTRACTION - SUPINE - WEIGHT	96	

EXERCISE Upper Extremity Strengthening and Range of Motion	EXERCISE NUMBER	NOTES
SCAPULAR PROTRACTION - SUPINE - ELASTIC BAND	97	
SCAPULAR PROTRACTION / TABLE PLANK	98	
CHEST PRESS – SEATED or STANDING - ELASTIC BAND	99	
CHEST PRESS – BALL, FLOOR or BENCH- WEIGHTS	100	
DOWEL PRESS – STANDING	101	
CHEST PRESS – STANDING or SEATED	102	
BENT OVER ROWS	103	
ROWS – PRONE	104	
ROWS - ELASTIC BAND	105	
WIDE ROWS - ELASTIC BAND	106	
LOW ROW – ELASTIC BAND	107	
HIGH ROW – ELASTIC BAND	108	
FLY'S – FLOOR - WEIGHT	109	
FLY'S – BALL or BENCH – WEIGHT	110	
WALL PUSH UPS	111	
WALL PUSH UP - BALL	112	
WALL PUSH UP - Triceps uneven	113	
WALL PUSH UP - Hands inverted	114	
WALL PUSH UP - Narrow	115	
WALL PUSH UP – Wide	116	
PUSH UPS - BALL	117	
PUSH UP - MODIFIED	118	
PUSH UP	119	
PUSH UP -DIAMOND	120	
PUSH UP – MODIFIED - BOSU - UNSTABLE	121	

EXERCISE Upper Extremity Strengthening and Range of Motion	EXERCISE NUMBER	NOTES
PUSH UP – BOSU - UNSTABLE	122	
PUSH UP – MODIFIED – INVERTED BOSU - UNSTABLE	123	
PUSH UP – INVERTED BOSU - UNSTABLE	124	

UPPER EXTREMITY - Range Of Motion > Isometric > Strength

Elbow Flexion/Extension

	_____ Reps _____ Sets _____ X Day _____ Hold		_____ Reps _____ Sets _____ X Day _____ Hold
1	Notes:	**2**	Notes:

Extension

Flexion

ELBOW FLEXION EXTENSION - SUPINE

Lie on your back and rest your elbow on a small rolled up towel. Bend at your elbow and then lower back down.

Flexion

Extension

ELBOW FLEXION / EXTENSION - GRAVITY ELIMINATED

Sit and hold your arm up with the help of your other arm. Bend and straighten your elbow.

Elbow Flexion (Biceps)

	_____ Reps _____ Sets _____ X Day _____ Hold		_____ Reps _____ Sets _____ X Day _____ Hold
3	Notes:	**4**	Notes:

BICEPS CURLS – ALTERNATING

Bend your elbow and move your forearm upwards. As you lower back down, begin bending the opposite elbow upwards.

BICEPS CURL - SELF FIXATION – ELASTIC BAND

Sit and hold an elastic band with one hand. Hold the other end of elastic band with the opposite hand and fixate hand on your knee. Slowly draw up your hand by bending at the elbow. Return to starting position and repeat.
*Can increase resistance by doubling band as shown.

	_____ Reps _____ Sets _____ X Day _____ Hold		_____ Reps _____ Sets _____ X Day _____ Hold
5	Notes:	**6**	Notes:

SEATED BICEPS CURLS - ALTERNATING

Sit in a chair and hold free weights on each thigh. Lift one side while bending at the elbow and squeezing bicep muscle. Perform on one side and then alternate to the other side.

SEATED BICEPS CURLS - BILATERAL

Sit in a chair and hold free weights on each thigh. Lift both sides while bending at the elbows and squeezing bicep muscles. Lower back down and repeat.

	_____ Reps _____ Sets _____ X Day _____ Hold		_____ Reps _____ Sets _____ X Day _____ Hold
7	Notes:	**8**	Notes:

CONCENTRATION CURLS – SITTING

Sit in a chair, lean slightly forward and hold a free weight with arm straight with elbow on inside of thigh. Bend elbow squeezing bicep muscle. Lower back down - repeat.

Starting Position

PREACHER CURL ON BALL

Lie on stomach over ball in crawling position. Hold weights in both hands with back of arms against ball. Lift both sides while bending at the elbows and squeezing bicep muscles. Lower back down - repeat.

_____ Reps _____ Sets _____ X Day _____ Hold	_____ Reps _____ Sets _____ X Day _____ Hold

9 | Notes:

10 | Notes:

BICEPS CURLS

Holding weights and keeping your arm at your side, draw up your hand by bending at the elbow squeezing bicep muscle. Keep your palm face up the entire time. Can perform set on one side and then other or alternate arms.

BICEPS CURLS - RADIOBRACHIALIS - HAMMER CURL

Holding weights and keeping your arm at your side, draw up your hand by bending at the elbow squeezing bicep muscle. Keep your wrist in a neutral position as shown above the entire time. Can perform set on one side and then other or alternate arms.

_____ Reps _____ Sets _____ X Day _____ Hold	_____ Reps _____ Sets _____ X Day _____ Hold

11 | Notes:

12 | Notes:

BICEPS CURLS - BRACHIALIS

Holding weights and keeping your arm at your side, draw up your hand by bending at the elbow squeezing bicep muscle. Keep your palm face down the entire time. Can perform set on one side and then other or alternate arms.

BICEPS CURLS – ROTATE OUTWARD

Holding weights and keeping your arm at your side, draw up your hand by bending at the elbow squeezing bicep muscle. Keep your palm face up the entire time. You can do this one arm at a time or bilateral.

	_____ Reps _____ Sets _____X Day _____Hold
13	Notes:

BICEPS CURLS – ONE ARM - ELASTIC BAND

In a standing position, step on the band with one leg. Keep your arm at your side holding an elastic band and draw up your hand by bending at the elbow squeezing bicep muscle. Keep your palm face up the entire time.

	_____ Reps _____ Sets _____X Day _____Hold
14	Notes:

BICEPS CURLS – BILATERAL - ELASTIC BAND

In a standing position, step on the band with both feet, shoulder width apart. Keep your arms at your side holding an elastic band and draw up your hands by bending at the elbows squeezing bicep muscles. Keep your palms facing upward the entire time.

	_____ Reps _____ Sets _____X Day _____Hold
15	Notes:

BICEPS CURLS - RADIOBRACHIALIS - HAMMER CURL – ONE ARM - ELASTIC BAND

In a standing position, step on the band with one leg. Keep your arm at your side holding an elastic band and draw up your hand by bending at the elbow squeezing bicep muscle. Keep your palm facing inward the entire time.

	_____ Reps _____ Sets _____X Day _____Hold
16	Notes:

BICEPS CURLS - RADIOBRACHIALIS - HAMMER CURL – BILATERAL - ELASTIC BAND

In a standing position, step on the band with both feet, shoulder width apart. Keep your arms at your side holding an elastic band and draw up your hands by bending at the elbows squeezing bicep muscles. Keep your palms facing inward the entire time.

	_____ Reps _____ Sets _____ X Day _____ Hold		_____ Reps _____ Sets _____ X Day _____ Hold
17	Notes:	18	Notes:

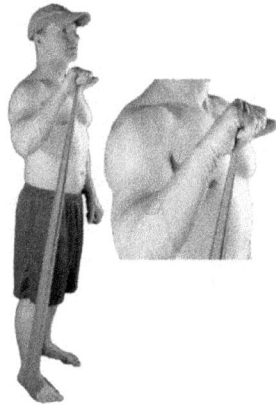

BICEPS CURLS – BRACHIALIS - ONE ARM - ELASTIC BAND

In a standing position, step on the band with one leg. Keep your arm at your side holding an elastic band and draw up your hand by bending at the elbow squeezing bicep muscle. Keep your palm face down the entire time.

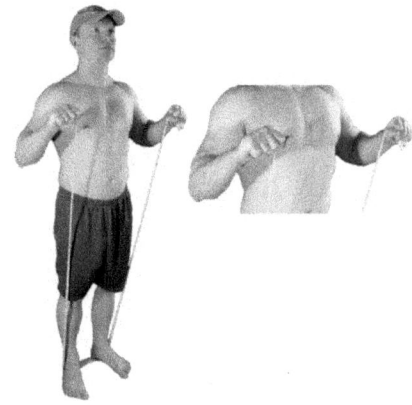

BICEPS CURL – BRACHIALIS – BILATERAL - ELASTIC BAND

In a standing position, step on the band with both feet, shoulder width apart. Keep your arms at your side holding an elastic band and draw up your hands by bending at the elbows squeezing bicep muscles. Keep your palms facing downward the entire time.

Elbow Extension (Triceps)

	_____ Reps _____ Sets _____ X Day _____ Hold		_____ Reps _____ Sets _____ X Day _____ Hold
19	Notes:	20	Notes:

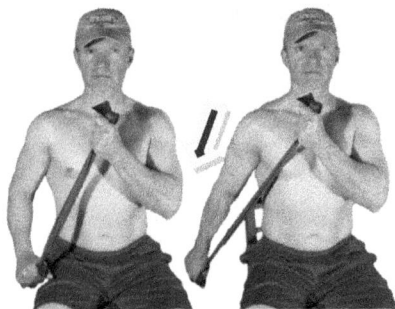

TRICEPS - SELF FIXATION - ELASTIC BAND

Hold an elastic band across your chest with the unaffected arm. Pull the band downward with the other arm so that the elbow goes from a bent position to a straightened position as shown.

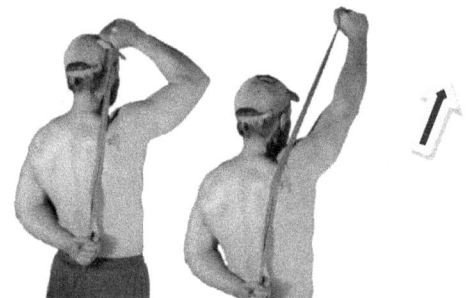

OVERHEAD TRICEPS - SELF FIXATION –SEATED OR STANDING - ELASTIC BAND

Hold an elastic band with one arm fixated behind back as shown and other hand behind head. Extend elbow with arm overhead and return to starting position.

	_____ Reps _____ Sets _____X Day _____Hold
21	**Notes:**

Starting

Position

TRICEP EXTENSION – SITTING OR STANDING - WEIGHT

Start with hand behind head holding free weight. Extend your elbow as shown. Maintain your upper arm in an upward direction and only bend and straighten at your elbow.
*Can hold the triceps area with opposite arm to stabilize.

	_____ Reps _____ Sets _____X Day _____Hold
22	**Notes:**

Starting

Position

TRICEP EXTENSION – SITTING OR STANDING – BILATERAL - WEIGHT

Start with hands behind head holding free weight Extend your elbows while holding a free weight in both hands. Maintain your upper arms in an upward direction and only bend and straighten at your elbows.

	_____ Reps _____ Sets _____X Day _____Hold
23	**Notes:**

Starting

Position

ELBOW EXTENSION - BALL

Lie on your back on ball. Extend your elbow as shown while holding a free weight in each hand. Maintain your upper arms in an upward direction and only bend and straighten at your elbows.

	_____ Reps _____ Sets _____X Day _____Hold
24	**Notes:**

ELBOW EXTENSION - SKULL CRUSHER - BALL

Lie on your back on ball with a free weight in each hand. Bend your elbows to lower the weight towards the side of your head and then extend arms straight up towards the ceiling.

	_____ Reps _____ Sets _____ X Day _____ Hold
25	Notes:

TRICEPS - ELASTIC BAND

Fixate the band at top of door. Start with your elbow bent and holding an elastic band as shown. Pull the elastic band downward as you extend your elbow. Keep your elbow by your side the entire time.

	_____ Reps _____ Sets _____ X Day _____ Hold
26	Notes:

TRICEPS - BENT OVER

Stand and bend over with either support or placing your unaffected arm on thigh for support. With your targeted arm and elbow at your side, extend your elbow as you straighten your arm as shown. Keep your elbow at your side and back flat the entire time.

	_____ Reps _____ Sets _____ X Day _____ Hold
27	Notes:

CHAIR DIPS / PUSH UPS

While sitting in a chair with arm rests, push yourself upawards so that you lift your buttocks of the chair and then lower down controlled back to normal seated position. *If you are unable to lift yourself up, you can perform "pressure releases" so that you simply push to take some weight off your buttocks.

	_____ Reps _____ Sets _____ X Day _____ Hold
28	Notes:

DIPS OFF CHAIR

Push yourself up to a straight elbow position as shown. Then lower your buttocks down towards the floor by bending your elbows.

Shoulder PENDULUMS

	_____ Reps _____ Sets _____ X Day _____ Hold		_____ Reps _____ Sets _____ X Day _____ Hold
29	Notes:	**30**	Notes:

PENDULUM SHOULDER FORWARD/BACK

Shift your body weight forward then back to allow your injured arm to swing forward and back freely. Your affected arm should be fully relaxed.

PENDULUM SHOULDER – SIDE TO SIDE

Shift your body weight side to side to allow your injured arm to swing side to side freely. Your affected arm should be fully relaxed.

	_____ Reps _____ Sets _____ X Day _____ Hold		_____ Reps _____ Sets _____ X Day _____ Hold
31	Notes:	**32**	Notes:

PENDULUM SHOULDER CIRCLES
Shift your body weight in circles to allow your injured arm to swing in circles freely. Your injured arm should be fully relaxed.
REVERSE PENDULUM SHOULDER CIRCLES
Shift your body weight into reverse circles to allow your injured arm to swing in circles freely. Your injured arm should be fully relaxed.

PENDULUMS - SUPINE

Lie on your back and straighten your arm towards the ceiling. Move your arm in small circles in a clockwise motion. After a few seconds, reverse the direction to a counterclockwise motion. Change directions every few seconds.

Shoulder Flexion

	_____ Reps _____ Sets _____ X Day _____ Hold		_____ Reps _____ Sets _____ X Day _____ Hold
33	Notes:	34	Notes:

ISOMETRIC FLEXION - Can use towel roll for comfort

Gently push your fist forward into a wall with your elbow bent. Hold for 5-10 seconds. Repeat.

Starting Position

SHOULDER FLEXION – SIDELYING - Can add weight

Lie on your side with arm at your side. Slowly raise the arm forward towards overhead and in front of your body.

	_____ Reps _____ Sets _____ X Day _____ Hold		_____ Reps _____ Sets _____ X Day _____ Hold
35	Notes:	36	Notes:

Starting Position

FLEXION – SUPINE - SINGLE OR BILATERAL

Lie on your back with your arm at your side. Slowly raise arm up and forward towards overhead.

Starting Position

FLEXION – SUPINE – SINGLE OR BILATERAL - WEIGHT

Lie on your back with your arm at your side. Holding a weight, slowly raise arm up and forward towards overhead.

	_____ Reps _____ Sets _____ X Day _____ Hold
37	**Notes:**

Starting Position

FLEXION – SUPINE - DOWEL

Lie on your back holding dowel with both hands. Slowly raise up and forward towards overhead. Return to starting position. Repeat.
*If you have an injury/weakness, allow your unaffected arm to perform most of the effort. Your affected arm should be partially relaxed.

	_____ Reps _____ Sets _____ X Day _____ Hold
38	**Notes:**

Starting Position

FLEXION – SUPINE - DOWEL – Add weight only if equal strength

Attach ankle weight to dowel. Lie on your back holding dowel with both hands. Slowly raise up and forward towards overhead. Return to starting position. Repeat.

	_____ Reps _____ Sets _____ X Day _____ Hold
39	**Notes:**

FLEXION - SELF FIXATION – ELASTIC BAND

Hold an elastic band in front and fixate unaffected arm straight by your side or on your leg. Pull the band upward towards the ceiling with your target arm.

	_____ Reps _____ Sets _____ X Day _____ Hold
40	**Notes:**

Starting Position

FLEXION – ELASTIC BAND

In a standing position, step on the band with one leg. Keep your arm at your side holding an elastic band and draw up your arm up in front of you keeping your elbow straight.

	_____ Reps _____ Sets _____ X Day _____ Hold
41	Notes:

FLEXION - STANDING - PALMS DOWN / OVERHAND DOWEL - Add weight only if equal strength

Hold a dowel/cane with both arms, palm down on both sides. Raise the dowel forward and up. (see #39/40) *Do not use weight if you have an injury/weakness. Allow your unaffected arm to perform most of the work. Your affected arm should be partially relaxed.

	_____ Reps _____ Sets _____ X Day _____ Hold
42	Notes:

FLEXION - STANDING - PALMS UP /UNDERHAND DOWEL - Add weight only if equal strength

Hold a dowel/cane with both arms and palms up on both sides. Raise the dowel forward and up. *Do not use weight if you have an injury/weakness. Allow your unaffected arm to perform most of the work. Your affected arm should be partially relaxed.

	_____ Reps _____ Sets _____ X Day _____ Hold
43	Notes:

FLEXION – PALMS FACING INWARD - Can remove weight BILATERAL or ALTERNATE ARMS.

Sit or stand with your arm at your side. Hold a free weight with your palm facing your side and your elbows straight. Raise up your arm forward as shown then return to starting position. Do not let your shoulder shrug upwards unless instructed to go over shoulder level height.

	_____ Reps _____ Sets _____ X Day _____ Hold
44	Notes:

FLEXION – PALMS DOWN - Can remove weight BILATERAL or ALTERNATE ARMS.

Sit or stand with your arm at your side. Hold a weight with your palm facing down and your elbows straight. Raise up your arm forward as shown then return to starting position. Do not let your shoulder shrug upwards unless instructed to go over shoulder height.

V Raises

	_____ Reps _____ Sets _____ X Day _____ Hold		_____ Reps _____ Sets _____ X Day _____ Hold
45	**Notes:**	**46**	**Notes:**

Starting
Position

V RAISE

Start with your arms down by your side, palms facing inward, thumbs up and your elbows straight. Raise up your arms in the form of a V to shoulder height as shown keeping elbows straight then return to starting position.

V RAISE – WEIGHTS

Holding free weights, start with your arms down by your side, palms facing inward and your elbows straight. Raise up your arms in the form of a V to shoulder height keeping elbows straight – return.

Shoulder Press

	_____ Reps _____ Sets _____ X Day _____ Hold		_____ Reps _____ Sets _____ X Day _____ Hold
47	**Notes:**	**48**	**Notes:**

Starting
Position

MILITARY PRESS – DOWEL- Add weight only if equal strength

Hold a dowel or cane at chest height. Slowly push the wand upwards towards the ceiling until your elbows become fully straightened. Return to the original position.

MILITARY PRESS - FREE WEIGHTS

Hold free weights at 90-degree angle as shown above.
Slowly push your arms upwards towards the ceiling until your elbows become fully straightened. Return to the original position.

Shoulder Extension

_____ Reps _____ Sets _____X Day _____Hold	_____ Reps _____ Sets _____X Day _____Hold
49 Notes:	**50** Notes:

ISOMETRIC EXTENSION - Can use towel roll for comfort

Gently push your bent elbow back into a wall. Hold for 5-10 seconds. Relax and repeat.

PRONE EXTENSION - EXERCISE BALL – Can add weights.

Lie face down over an exercise ball with your elbows straight and along the side of your body. Slowly raise your arms upward along your side and then return to original position.

_____ Reps _____ Sets _____X Day _____Hold	_____ Reps _____ Sets _____X Day _____Hold
51 Notes:	**52** Notes:

SHOULDER EXTENSION - STANDING

Start with arms by your side. Draw your arm back behind your waist. Keep your elbows straight.

SHOULDER EXTENSION - STANDING - WEIGHTS

Hold a weight by your side and draw your arm back. Keep your elbows straight.

	_____ Reps _____ Sets _____ X Day _____ Hold
53	Notes:

EXTENSION – STANDING – DOWEL - Add weight only if equal strength

Hold a dowel or cane behind your back with both arms. Draw your arms back.

	_____ Reps _____ Sets _____ X Day _____ Hold
54	Notes:

EXTENSION - SELF FIXATION - ELASTIC BAND

Hold an elastic band out in front of you with your fixated arm. Pull the band downward towards the ground and backwards with your target arm.

	_____ Reps _____ Sets _____ X Day _____ Hold
55	Notes:

EXTENSION - ELASTIC BAND

Fixate the end of an elastic band at top of door. Hold the elastic band in front of you with your elbows straight. Slowly pull the band down and back towards your side.

	_____ Reps _____ Sets _____ X Day _____ Hold
56	Notes:

EXTENSION - BILATERAL - ELASTIC BAND

Fixate the middle of an elastic band at top of door. Hold the elastic band with both arms in front of you with your elbows straight. Slowly pull the band downwards and back towards your side.

Shoulder Internal Rotation (IR)

	_____ Reps _____ Sets _____ X Day _____ Hold		_____ Reps _____ Sets _____ X Day _____ Hold
57	Notes:	**58**	Notes:

INTERNAL ROTATION – ISOMETRIC - Can use towel roll for comfort

Press your hand into a wall using the palm side of your hand and hold. Maintain a bent elbow the entire time.

INTERNAL ROTATION - ISOMETRIC- ELEVATED - Can use towel roll for comfort

Push the front of your hand into a wall with your elbow bent and arm elevated and hold.

	_____ Reps _____ Sets _____ X Day _____ Hold		_____ Reps _____ Sets _____ X Day _____ Hold
59	Notes:	**60**	Notes:

INTERNAL ROTATION - SIDELYING

Lie on your side with your shoulder flexed to 90 degrees and elbow bent and rested on the table/bed/matt. Your forearm should be pointing up towards the ceiling. Allow your forearm to lower toward the table as shown. Place a rolled-up towel under your elbow if needed.

INTERNAL ROTATION - ELASTIC BAND

Hold an elastic band at your side with your elbow bent. Start with your hand away from your stomach and then pull the band towards your stomach. Keep your elbow near your side the entire time.

	_____ Reps _____ Sets _____ X Day _____ Hold
61	Notes:

INTERNAL / EXTERNAL ROTATION - STANDING – DOWEL
Add weight only if equal strength

Stand and hold a dowel/cane with both hands keeping your elbows bent. Move your arms and dowel/cane side-to-side. _If you have an injury/weakness, the affected arm should be partially relaxed while your unaffected arm performs most of the effort._

	_____ Reps _____ Sets _____ X Day _____ Hold
62	Notes:

Starting Position

INTERNAL ROTATION – DOWEL - Add weight only if equal strength

While holding a dowel/cane behind your back, slowly pull the wand up.

Shoulder External Rotation (ER)

	_____ Reps _____ Sets _____ X Day _____ Hold
63	Notes:

EXTERNAL ROTATION - ISOMETRIC – Can use towel roll for comfort

Gently press your hand into a wall using the back side of your hand. Maintain a bent elbow the entire time.

	_____ Reps _____ Sets _____ X Day _____ Hold
64	Notes:

EXTERNAL ROTATION - ISOMETRIC – ELEVATED - Can use towel roll for comfort

Gently push the back of your hand/arm into a wall with your arm elevated.

_____ Reps _____ Sets _____X Day _____Hold

65	Notes:

Starting Position

EXTERNAL ROTATION WITH TOWEL - SIDELYING

Lie on your side with your elbow bent to 90 degrees. Place a rolled-up towel between your arm and the side your body as shown. Squeeze your shoulder blade back and rotate arm up and hold this position. Slowly rotate back to original position and repeat.

_____ Reps _____ Sets _____X Day _____Hold

66	Notes:

Starting Position

EXTERNAL ROTATION – 90/90 - WEIGHTS

Hold weights with elbows bent to 90 degrees and away from your side. Rotate your shoulders back so that the palms of your hands face forward and then return as shown.

_____ Reps _____ Sets _____X Day _____Hold

67	Notes:

EXTERNAL ROTATION - BILATERAL - ELASTIC BAND
Can put a towel between side and elbow (see #68)

Hold an elastic band with your elbows bent, pull your hands away from your stomach area. Keep your elbows near the side of your body.

_____ Reps _____ Sets _____X Day _____Hold

68	Notes:

EXTERNAL ROTATION - ELASTIC BAND – Can add roll between side and arm

Fixate an elastic band to the door at elbow height. Hold the other end of the band at your side with your elbow bent. Start with your hand near your stomach and then pull the band away. Keep your elbow at your side the entire time.

Shoulder Adduction (ADD)

	_____ Reps _____ Sets _____X Day _____Hold		_____ Reps _____ Sets _____X Day _____Hold
69	**Notes:**	**70**	**Notes:**

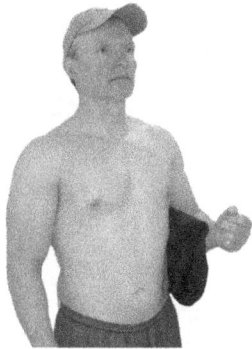

ADDUCTION – ISOMETRIC - Can use towel roll for comfort

Place a towel roll between your bent elbow and body. Gently push your elbow into the side of your body.

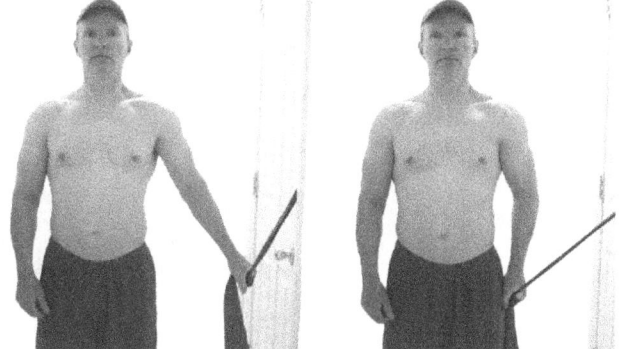

ADDUCTION - ELASTIC BAND

Fixate an elastic band to the door and hold the other end of the band away from your side. Pull the band towards your side keeping your elbow straight.

Shoulder Abduction (ABD)

	_____ Reps _____ Sets _____X Day _____Hold		_____ Reps _____ Sets _____X Day _____Hold
71	**Notes:**	**72**	**Notes:**

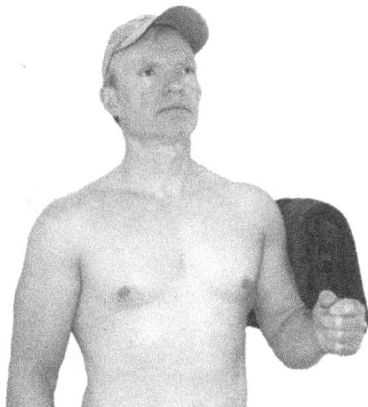

ABDUCTION – ISOMETRIC - Can use towel roll for comfort

Gently push your elbow out to the side into a wall with your elbow bent.

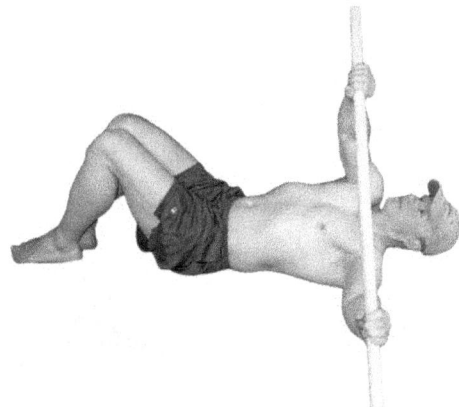

HORIZONTAL ABDUCTION - DOWEL

Lie on your back holding a dowel/cane straight up towards the ceiling with your elbows straight. Bring your arms and wand to the side and then towards the other.

	_____ Reps _____ Sets _____X Day _____Hold
73	Notes:

Starting

Position

HORIZONTAL ABDUCTION/ADDUCTTION - SUPINE
Lie on your back with arm straight up in front of your body. Slowly lower your arm out towards the side. Return to original position.

	_____ Reps _____ Sets _____X Day _____Hold
74	Notes:

Starting

Position

HORIZONTAL ABDUCTION/ADDUCTTION - SUPINE - WEIGHT

Hold a weight. Lie on your back with arm straight up in front of your body. Slowly lower your arm out towards the side. Return to original position

	_____ Reps _____ Sets _____X Day _____Hold
75	Notes:

Starting

Position

ABDUCTION - SIDELYING - Can add weight

Lie on your side with arm at your side. Slowly raise the target arm up towards head and away from your side.

	_____ Reps _____ Sets _____X Day _____Hold
76	Notes:

Starting

Position

HORIZONTAL ABDUCTION - SIDELYING - Can add weight

Lie on your side with arm out in front of your body. Slowly raise up the arm overhead towards the ceiling.

	_____ Reps _____ Sets _____X Day _____Hold
77	Notes:

ABDUCTION – WEIGHT – Can do without a weight

Hold a weight with your affected arm at your side. Keeping your elbow straight, raise up your arm to the side.

	_____ Reps _____ Sets _____X Day _____Hold
78	Notes:

ABDUCTION – ELASTIC BAND

Fixate an elastic band under a door and hold band with hand farthest away from door at your side. Keeping your elbow straight, raise up your arm to the side.

	_____ Reps _____ Sets _____X Day _____Hold
79	Notes:

HORIZONTAL ABDUCTION – BILATERAL - ELASTIC BAND

Hold an elastic band in both hands with your elbows straight in front of your body. Slowly pull your arms apart towards the sides.

	_____ Reps _____ Sets _____X Day _____Hold
80	Notes:

90/90 ABDUCTION - WEIGHT

Hold weights at your side with elbows bent to 90 degrees. Raise up your elbows away from your side while maintaining your elbows bent at 90 degrees.

Lateral/Frontal Raise

	_____ Reps _____ Sets _____X Day _____Hold
81	Notes:

	_____ Reps _____ Sets _____X Day _____Hold
82	Notes:

LATERAL RAISES

Hold weights at your side with arms straight. Raise up your elbows away from your side while keeping your elbow straight the entire time.

LATERAL RAISES – LEAN FORWARD

Bend slightly at the waist holding weights slightly in front. Raise up your elbows away from your side squeezing shoulder blades together.

	_____ Reps _____ Sets _____X Day _____Hold
83	Notes:

	_____ Reps _____ Sets _____X Day _____Hold
84	Notes:

LATERAL RAISES – LEAN FORWARD - ARM ROTATION

Bend slightly at the waist holding weights slightly in front as shown palms facing your body. Raise up your elbows away from your side squeezing shoulder blades together.

FRONTAL RAISE – WEIGHTS – Can do without weights

Hold weights at your side with arms straight. Slowly raise your arms in front of of your body.

Upright Rows

	_____ Reps _____ Sets _____X Day _____Hold		_____ Reps _____ Sets _____X Day _____Hold
85	Notes:	86	Notes:

Starting
Position

UPRIGHT ROW – WEIGHTS - Can use kettle bell

Hold weights or kettlebell with both hands at waist height. Lift the weights to chest height as you bend at your elbows.

Starting
Position

UPRIGHT ROW – ELASTIC BAND

Stand on an elastic band with either one or both feet. Hold band at waist height and raise it up to chest height as you bend at your elbows.

Shoulder Shrugs & Rolls

	_____ Reps _____ Sets _____X Day _____Hold		_____ Reps _____ Sets _____X Day _____Hold
87	Notes:	88	Notes:

SHRUGS

Raise your shoulders upward towards your ears as shown. Shrug both shoulders at the same time.

Starting
Position

SHRUGS - WEIGHTS

Hold weights in both hands with arms straight. Raise your shoulders upward towards your ears. Shrug both shoulders at the same time.

	____ Reps ____ Sets ____X Day ____Hold			____ Reps ____ Sets ____X Day ____Hold
89	Notes:		90	Notes:

SHOULDER ROLLS

Move your shoulders in a circular pattern so that your are moving in an up, back and down direction. Perform small circles if needed for comfort.
Complete one set and then reverse direction

SHOULDER ROLLS - WEIGHTS

Hold weights in both or one hand. Move your shoulders in a circular pattern so that your are moving in an up, back and down direction.
Complete one set and then reverse direction

Scapular Retraction

	____ Reps ____ Sets ____X Day ____Hold			____ Reps ____ Sets ____X Day ____Hold
91	Notes:		92	Notes:

SCAPULAR RETRACTIONS - BILATERAL

Draw your shoulder blades back and down.

SCAPULAR RETRACTION – SINGLE ARM

With your arm raised up and elbow bent, draw your shoulder blade back and down.

	_____ Reps _____ Sets _____ X Day _____ Hold
93	Notes:

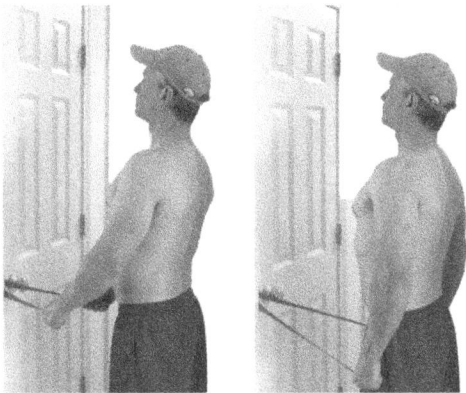

ELASTIC BAND SCAPULAR RETRACTIONS WITH MINI SHOULDER EXTENSIONS

Fixate an elastic band to the door and hold with both arms in front of you with your elbows straight. Slowly squeeze your shoulder blades together as you pull the band back. Be sure your shoulders do not rise up.

	_____ Reps _____ Sets _____ X Day _____ Hold
94	Notes:

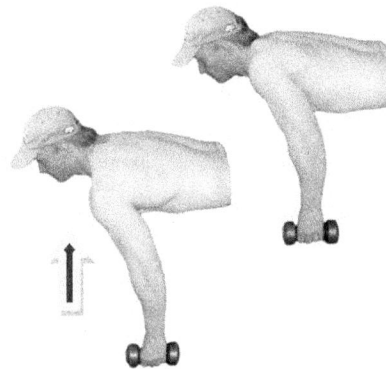

PRONE RETRACTION – Can do without weight

Lie face down with your elbows straight. Slowly draw your shoulder blade back towards your spine. Your whole arm should rise including your shoulder blade upward as shown. Your elbow should be straight the entire time.

Scapular Protraction

	_____ Reps _____ Sets _____ X Day _____ Hold
95	Notes:

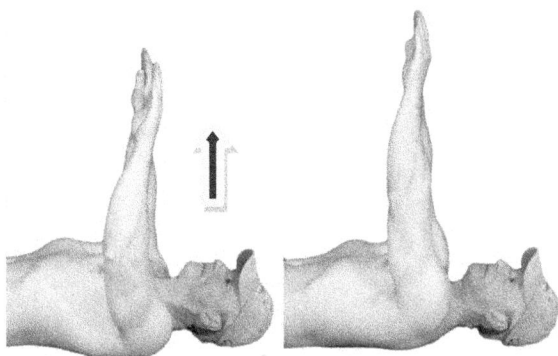

SCAPULAR PROTRACTION - SUPINE - BILATERAL

Lie on your back with your arms extended out in front of your body and towards the ceiling. While keeping your elbows straight, protract your shoulders reaching forward towards the ceiling. Keep your elbows straight the entire time.

	_____ Reps _____ Sets _____ X Day _____ Hold
96	Notes:

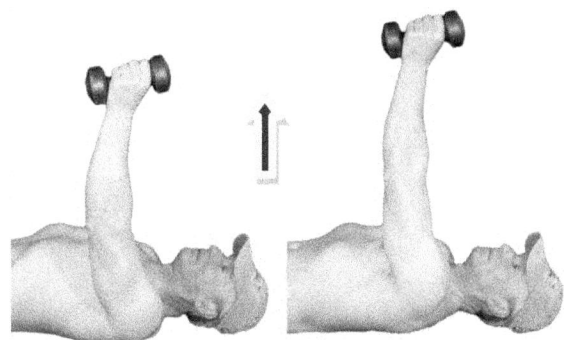

SCAPULAR PROTRACTION - SUPINE - WEIGHT

Lie on your back holding a weight with your arm extended out in front of your body and towards the ceiling. While keeping your elbows straight, protract your shoulders reaching forward towards the ceiling. Keep your elbows straight the entire time.

	_____ Reps _____ Sets _____ X Day _____ Hold		_____ Reps _____ Sets _____ X Day _____ Hold
97	Notes:	98	Notes:

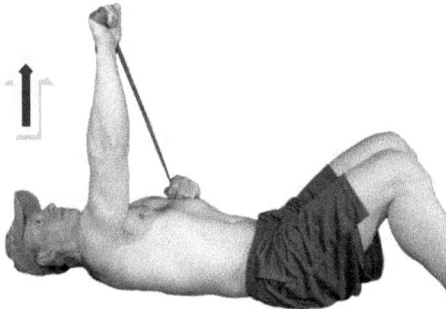

SCAPULAR PROTRACTION - SUPINE - ELASTIC BAND

Lie on your back and hold elastic band in both hands. Bend the unaffected arm to fixate the band. Extend the target arm out in front of your body and straight up towards the ceiling. While keeping your elbows straight, protract your shoulder blade forward towards the ceiling. Keep your elbows straight the entire time.

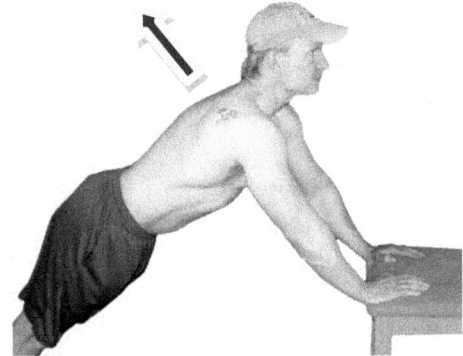

SCAPULAR PROTRACTION / TABLE PLANK

Start in a push up position on your hands and leaning up against a table or countertop as shown. Maintain this position as you protract your shoulder blades forward to raise your body upward a few inches. Return to original position.
*Progress by standing further away from the table.

Chest Press

	_____ Reps _____ Sets _____ X Day _____ Hold		_____ Reps _____ Sets _____ X Day _____ Hold
99	Notes:	100	Notes:

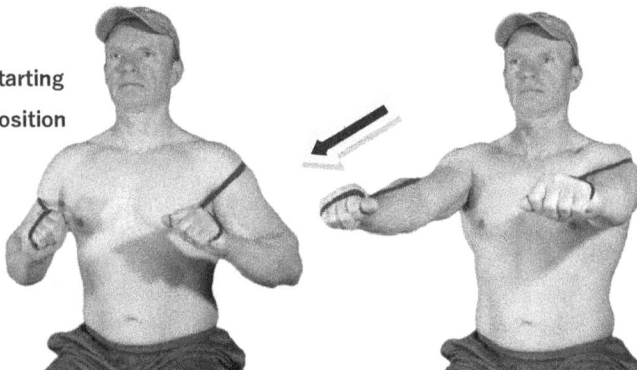

CHEST PRESS – SEATED or STANDING - ELASTIC BAND

Hold elastic band with both hands at your side and elbows bent with band wrapped around body or chair. Push the band out in front of your body as you straighten your elbows.

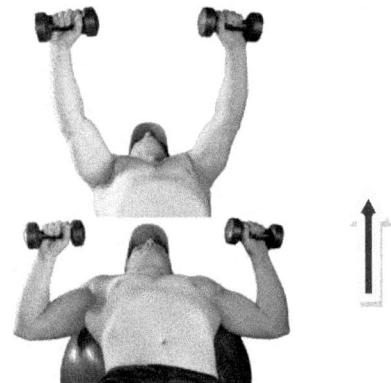

CHEST PRESS – BALL, FLOOR or BENCH- WEIGHTS

Lie on your back with your elbows bent. Slowly raise up your arms towards the ceiling while extending your elbows straight up above your head.

	_____ Reps _____ Sets _____X Day _____Hold
101	**Notes:**

Starting
Position

DOWEL PRESS – STANDING – Add weight only if equal strength

Hold a dowel/cane at chest height. Slowly push the dowel outwards in front of your body so that your elbows become fully straightened. Return to the original position.

	_____ Reps _____ Sets _____X Day _____Hold
102	**Notes:**

Starting
Position

CHEST PRESS – STANDING or SEATED

Hold weights in both hands with your arms at your side and elbows bent. Push your arms out in front of your body as you straighten your elbows.

Rows

	_____ Reps _____ Sets _____X Day _____Hold
103	**Notes:**

BENT OVER ROWS

Stand, bend over and support yourself with the unaffected arm. Slowly draw up your target arm as you bend your elbow. Keep your back flat the entire time.

	_____ Reps _____ Sets _____X Day _____Hold
104	**Notes:**

ROWS – PRONE – On bed or table

Lie face down with your elbows straight, slowly raise your arms upward while bending your elbows.

	_____ Reps _____ Sets _____X Day _____Hold			
105	Notes:			

ROWS - ELASTIC BAND

Fixate the elastic band in the door at elbow level. Hold the elastic band with both hands, draw back the band as you bend your elbows. Keep your elbows near the side of your body.

	_____ Reps _____ Sets _____X Day _____Hold			
106	Notes:			

WIDE ROWS - ELASTIC BAND

Fixate the elastic band in the door and hold the band with both hands. Draw back the band as you bend your elbows squeezing shoulder blades together. Keep your arms about 90 degrees away from the side of your body.

	_____ Reps _____ Sets _____X Day _____Hold			
107	Notes:			

LOW ROW – ELASTIC BAND

Fixate the elastic band in the door below elbow level. Hold the elastic band with both hands, draw back the band as you bend your elbows. Keep your elbows near the side of your body.

	_____ Reps _____ Sets _____X Day _____Hold			
108	Notes:			

HIGH ROW – ELASTIC BAND

Fixate the elastic band at the top of the door. Hold the elastic band with both hands, draw back the band as you bend your elbows. Keep your elbows near the side of your body.

Flys

109	_____ Reps _____ Sets _____ X Day _____ Hold		110	_____ Reps _____ Sets _____ X Day _____ Hold
	Notes:			Notes:

Starting
Position

FLY'S – FLOOR - WEIGHT

Holding weights, lie on your back with your arms horizontally out to the side. Bring your arms up and forward towards the ceiling. Lower your arms back down to the original position. Your elbows should be partially bent the entire time.

FLY'S – BALL or BENCH – WEIGHT

Holding weights, lie on your back on a ball with your arms horizontally out to the side. Bring your arms up and forward towards the ceiling. Lower your arms back down to the original position with elbows partially bent the entire time.

Wall pushups – To progress, move feet further away from wall

111	_____ Reps _____ Sets _____ X Day _____ Hold		112	_____ Reps _____ Sets _____ X Day _____ Hold
	Notes:			Notes:

WALL PUSH UPS

Place your arms out in front of you with your elbows straight so that your hands just reach the wall. Bend your elbows slowly to bring your chest closer to the wall. Straighten your arms pushing your body away from wall. Maintain your feet planted on the ground the entire time.

WALL PUSH UP - BALL

Place a ball on a wall while holding the ball with both hands as shown. Bend your elbows slowly to bring your chest closer to the wall and then straighten your arms pushing your body away from wall. Maintain your feet planted on the ground the entire time.

	_____ Reps _____ Sets _____X Day _____Hold
113	Notes:

WALL PUSH UP - Triceps uneven

Place your arms out in front of you with your elbows straight in an uneven position so that your hands just reach the wall. Bend your elbows slowly to bring your chest closer to the wall and then straighten your arms pushing your body away from wall. Maintain your feet planted on the ground the entire time.

	_____ Reps _____ Sets _____X Day _____Hold
114	Notes:

WALL PUSH UP – Hands inverted

Place your arms out in front of you with your elbows straight and hands inverted just reaching the wall. Bend your elbows slowly to bring your chest closer to the wall and then straighten your arms pushing your body away from wall. Maintain your feet planted on the ground the entire time.

	_____ Reps _____ Sets _____X Day _____Hold
115	Notes:

WALL PUSH UP - Narrow

Place your arms out in front of you with your elbows straight and hands close togther just reaching the wall. Bend your elbows slowly to bring your chest closer to the wall and then straighten your arms pushing your body away from wall. Maintain your feet planted on the ground the entire time.

	_____ Reps _____ Sets _____X Day _____Hold
116	Notes:

WALL PUSH UP – Wide

Place your arms out in front of you with your elbows straight and your arms and hands far apart just reaching the wall. Bend your elbows slowly to bring your chest closer to the wall and then straighten your arms pushing your body away from wall. Maintain your feet planted on the ground the entire time.

Push ups

	_____ Reps _____ Sets _____X Day _____Hold		_____ Reps _____ Sets _____X Day _____Hold
117	**Notes:**	**118**	**Notes:**

Starting

Position

PUSH UPS - BALL

Start in a kneeling position with an exercise ball in front of you. Slowly walk yourself out with your arms so that the ball is positioned under your legs. Then perform push ups. *Progress by moving ball back towards thighs

PUSH UP - MODIFIED

Lie face down and use your arms and push yourself up. Keep your knees in contact with the floor and maintain a straight back the entire time.

	_____ Reps _____ Sets _____X Day _____Hold		_____ Reps _____ Sets _____X Day _____Hold
119	**Notes:**	**120**	**Notes:**

Starting

Position

PUSH UP

Lie face down, use your arms and push yourself. Keep your toes in contact with the floor and maintain a straight back the entire time.

PUSH UP -DIAMOND

Lie face down and place your hands on the floor in the shape of a diamond with your thumbs and index fingers.
Use your arms and push yourself up.. Keep your toes in contact with the floor and maintain a straight back the entire time.

_____ Reps _____ Sets _____ X Day _____ Hold	_____ Reps _____ Sets _____ X Day _____ Hold
121 Notes:	**122** Notes:

PUSH UP – MODIFIED - BOSU - UNSTABLE

Perform push-ups with your hands on a Bosu. Keep your knees in contact with the floor and maintain a straight back the entire time.

PUSH UP – BOSU - UNSTABLE

Perform push-ups with your hands on top of a Bosu. Keep your toes in contact with the floor and maintain a straight back the entire time.

_____ Reps _____ Sets _____ X Day _____ Hold	_____ Reps _____ Sets _____ X Day _____ Hold
123 Notes:	**124** Notes:

PUSH UP – MODIFIED – INVERTED BOSU - UNSTABLE

Perform push-ups while holding an inverted Bosu. Try and maintain the Bosu platform as level as you can. Keep your knees in contact with the floor and maintain a straight back the entire time.

PUSH UP – INVERTED BOSU - UNSTABLE

Perform push-ups while holding an inverted Bosu. Try and maintain the Bosu platform as level as you can. Keep your toes in contact with the floor and maintain a straight back the entire time.

BALANCE – CORE – STANDING LE STRENGTH

Basics
- Requires LE strengthening for progression
- Perform exercises 2-3x a week
- Should be performed at beginning of exercise routine or can be the main exercise routine for endurance with increased repetitions or strength with resistance.

Duration, Frequency, Intensity, Sets and Reps
- Balance – 1 set, 2-4 repetitions for hold of 5-60 seconds
- Endurance – Less than 30 second rests in between sets
  - Static - 1 set, 5-10 repetitions as tolerated
  - Dynamic – 1 set, 3-10 reps for 10-30+ second hold as tolerated
- Strengthening – Add resistance with bands or weights (*see Strengthening for more information*)
  - Static – 2-3 sets, 3-12 reps – slow controlled movements
  - Dynamic – 1-3 sets, 2-4 reps

Static Balance Progression:
1. Bilateral – Both feet on the ground
2. Unilateral – One foot on the ground
3. Arm Movement – Overhead, can do arm exercises (*See Arm Strengthening for exercises*)
4. Trunk rotation – Rotate with or without arm movement
5. Eyes Shut (lack of visual cues – sensory removal)
6. Head Turns, hand/eye tracking, shifting focal point (vestibular – sensory alteration)
7. Reading (coordination)
8. Unstable – progression
Repeat above on unstable surface such as balance pad, pillow, balance disc or Bosu.

Decrease Base of Support (BOS) Progression:
- Wide BOS
- Narrow Bos
- Staggered/Split Stance/Semi-tandem
- Tandem Stance
- Single Leg Stance

SOLID GROUND:
1. Support: Hold onto chair, counter, sink or another stationary object.
2. No Support: Stand next to stable surface if needed for security.
   - Can start with 1-2 hands and as you become more stable, decrease the number of fingers used for support. For example, take away the thumb and hold with 4 fingers, 3 fingers, 2 fingers, 1 finger and then without support.
3. Resistance: Add ankle weights on use elastic band for resistance

UNSTABLE SURFACE: Balance pad, Bosu, Half foam roll, Pillow or Other unstable surface
1. Support: Hold onto chair, counter or another stationary object.
2. No Support: Stand next to stable surface if needed for security.
   - Can start with 1-2 hands and as you become more stable, decrease the number of fingers used for support. For example, take away the thumb and hold with 4 fingers, 3 fingers, 2 fingers, 1 finger and then without support.
3. Resistance: Add ankle weights on use elastic band for resistance

Peripheral Neuropathy Caution Balancing on Uneven Surface	• Peripheral neuropathy can be a side effect of diabetes or may be as a result of damage to the peripheral nerves. These nerves carry information from the brain to other parts of the body. • Feet or lower extremity – Caution standing on uneven surface, such as a Bosu ball or balance pads due to decreased sensation in feet. Increased risk of falling. • Hands – Caution with holding dumbbells or grasping resistance bands.

Balance

EXERCISE Balance	EXERCISE NUMBER	NOTES
WIDE BOS DECREASING TO NARROW BOS	1	
NARROW BOS	2	
ARM MOVEMENT	3	
TRUNK ROTATION	4	
EYES SHUTS	5	
HEAD TURNS	6	
READING ALOUD	7	
BALANCE PAD	8	
SPLIT STANCE – SEMI TANDEM	9	
SPLIT STANCE - *Progression*	10	
TANDEM- SHARPENED ROMBERG STANCE	11	
TANDEM STANCE - Progression	12	
SINGLE LEG STANCE (SLS)	13	
SINGLE LEG STANCE (SLS) - *Progression*	14	
SLS – LEG FORWARD	15	
SLS – LEG BACKWARDS	16	
SLS – LEG FORWARD / OPPOSITE ARM UP	17	
SLS – LEG BACKWARDS / OPPOSITE ARM UP	18	
SLS - REACH FORWARD	19	
SLS - REACH TWIST	20	
SINGLE LEG TOE TAP	21	
SINGLE LEG STANCE - CLOCKS	22	
BALL ROLLS - HEEL TOE	23	
BALL ROLLS - LATERAL	24	
SQUAT	25	
SIT TO STAND	26	

Balance

EXERCISE	EXERCISE NUMBER	NOTES
SQUATS – WALL WITH BALL	27	
SQUATS WITH WEIGHTS	28	
MINI SQUAT - UNSTABLE SUPPORT - FOAM PAD	29	
SQUATS - SINGLE LEG	30	
SIDE TO SIDE WEIGHT SHIFT	31	
FORWARD AND BACKWARDS WEIGHT SHIFTS	32	
SPLIT STANCE WEIGHT SHIFT SIDE TO SIDE	33	
SPLIT STANCE WEIGHT SHIFT FORWARD AND BACKWARDS	34	
WALL FALLS - FORWARD - BALANCE DRILL	35	
WALL FALLS - LATERAL - BALANCE DRILL	36	
WALL FALLS - BACKWARDS - BALANCE DRILL	37	
WALL FALLS - SINGLE LEG - FORWARD - BALANCE DRILL	38	
WALL FALLS - SINGLE LEG - LATERAL - BALANCE DRILL	39	
WALL FALLS - SINGLE LEG - MEDIAL - BALANCE DRILL	40	
WALL FALLS - SINGLE LEG - BACKWARDS - BALANCE DRILL	41	
FALL LATERAL - STEP RECOVERY	42	
FALL FORWARD - STEP RECOVERY	43	
FALL BACKWARD - STEP RECOVERY	44	
TOE TAP ABDUCTION	45	
HIP ABDUCTION - STANDING	46	
HIP EXTENSION – STANDING	47	
HIP FLEXION - STANDING – STRAIGHT LEG RAISE	48	
HIP / KNEE FLEXION - SINGLE LEG	49	
STANDING MARCHING	50	

Balance

EXERCISE Balance	EXERCISE NUMBER	NOTES
HAMSTRING CURL	51	
TOE RAISES	52	
TOE RAISES IR AND ER	53	
ONE LEGGED TOE RAISE	54	
SINGLE LEG BALANCE FORWARD	55	
SINGLE LEG BALANCE LATERAL	56	
SINGLE LEG BALANCE RETRO	57	
SINGLE LEG STANCE RETROLATERAL	58	
SQUAT	59	
SINGLE LEG SQUAT	60	
LUNGE – STATIC	61	
LUNGE FORWARD/BACKWARD	62	
FOUR CORNER MARCHING IN PLACE	63	
FOUR CORNER MARCHING IN PLACE WITH HEAD TURNS	64	
WALKING ON HEELS FORWARD AND BACKWARDS	65	
WALKING ON TOES FORWARD AND BACKWARDS	66	
TANDEM STANCE AND WALK – FORWARD AND BACKWARDS	67	
RUNNING MAN	68	
HOP STICK - FORWARD	69	
HOP STICK - BACKWARDS	70	
MINI LATERAL LUNGE	71	
SIDE STEPPING	72	
HOP STICK - LATERAL	73	
SINGLE LEG DEAD LIFT	74	

Balance

EXERCISE	EXERCISE NUMBER	NOTES
Balance		
CONE TAPS - SINGLE LEG STANCE	75	
CONE TAPS - SINGLE LEG STANCE - UNSTABLE	76	
FIGURE 8 AROUND CONES	77	
FIGURE 8 AROUND CONES – FOOT OR HAND TAP	78	
BALANCE DOUBLE LEG STANCE - WIDE	79	
BALANCE DOUBLE LEG STANCE - NARROW	80	
TANDEM STANCE	81	
TANDEM WALK	82	
SINGLE LEG STANCE - ABDUCTION	83	
SINGLE LEG STANCE - ABDUCTION	84	
SINGLE LEG STANCE – FORWARD KICK	85	
SINGLE LEG STANCE – HAMSTRING CURL	86	
SINGLE LEG SQUAT – LEG FORWARD	87	
SINGLE LEG SQUAT – LEG BACKWARDS	88	
TOE TAP OR HEEL PLACEMENT	89	
PULL UP FOOT TOUCHES ON STEP	90	
ALTERNATING SUSTAINED FOOT TOUCHES ON STEP	91	
STEP UP AND OVER	92	
FORWARD SWING THROUGH STEP	93	
SIDE STEPPING - *REPEAT STEPS 89-93 from a side approach.*	94	

BALANCE PROGRESSION- STATIC – See WARNING above Re: Peripheral Neuropathy

Hip Width/Narrow Stance >>>>> Staggered Stance >>>>> Tandem Stance >>>>> Single-Leg Stance

1. Hold onto a chair, counter or other steady object.
2. Continue steps 2-8 holding on to a sturdy object.
3. Can start with 1-2 hands and as you become more stable, decrease the number of fingers used for support. For example, take away the thumb and hold with 4 fingers, 3 fingers, 2 fingers, 1 finger and then without support.
4. When feeling comfortable, take away support staying close to object for security
5. When able to complete with decreased support, add balance pad or unstable surface completing 2-8 as above.

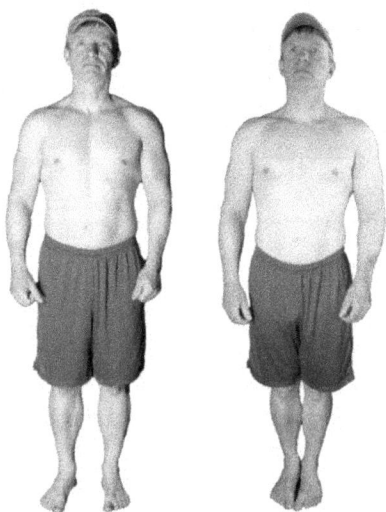

HIP WIDTH OR WIDE BASE OF SUPPORT (BOS) >
NARROW BASE OF SUPPORT (BOS)

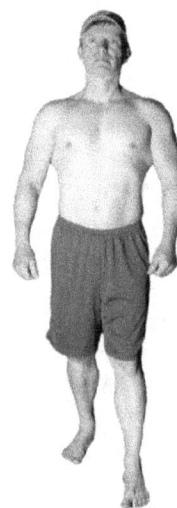

STAGGERED STANCE – SPLIT STANCE

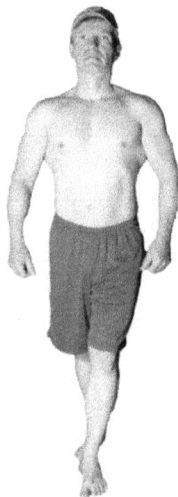

TANDEM STANCE

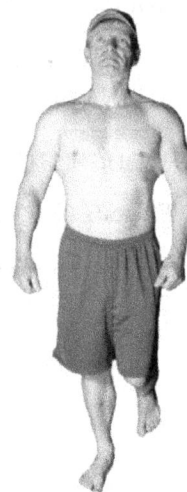

SINGLE LEG STANCE

1	_____ Reps _____ Sets _____X Day _____Hold **Notes:**

2	_____ Reps _____ Sets _____X Day _____Hold **Notes:**

WIDE BOS DECREASING TO NARROW BOS

Continue steps 2-8 holding on to a sturdy object and then progress with decreased support as outlined above.

NARROW BOS

Stand with your feet together Count to 10. Increase time up to 60 seconds as tolerated maintaining your balance in this position.

3	_____ Reps _____ Sets _____X Day _____Hold **Notes:**

4	_____ Reps _____ Sets _____X Day _____Hold **Notes:**

ARM MOVEMENT

Examples:
- Throw ball up in arm and catch
- Play catch with partner
- Reach hands above head and then down by side
- Do standing arm exercises (*See Arm Strengthening for examples*)

TRUNK ROTATION – reach side to side

Examples:
- Reach side to side within BOS
- Reach side to side and forward out of BOS

Balance

_____ Reps _____ Sets _____ X Day _____ Hold	_____ Reps _____ Sets _____ X Day _____ Hold
5 Notes:	**6** Notes:

EYES SHUTS - Lack of visual cues – *Sensory Removal*

Stand with eyes shut and count to 10. Increase time up to 60 seconds as tolerated.

HEAD TURNS - Vestibular – *Sensory Alteration*

Examples:
- Turn head slowly from side to side
- Move head up and down slowly
- Put one finger out in front of face at arm's length moving in outward/inward direction and move head to follow with eyes. Slow hand tracking.
- Shift focal point to different objects in the room
- *Can add head turns with eyes closed*

_____ Reps _____ Sets _____ X Day _____ Hold	_____ Reps _____ Sets _____ X Day _____ Hold
7 Notes:	**8** Notes:

READING ALOUD - *Coordination / Cognitive Task*

Hold reading material, such as a book, paper, tablet, or magazine in one or both hands. Read out loud and progress to moving your head and the object on occasion to the side or up/down.

BALANCE PAD or another unstable surface

Place balance pad, Bosu, pillow or other unstable surface by a chair or counter for support. Stand on the pad.

****REPEAT STEPS 2-8 on unstable surface****

	_____ Reps _____ Sets _____X Day _____Hold		_____ Reps _____ Sets _____X Day _____Hold
9	Notes:	10	Notes:

SPLIT STANCE – SEMI TANDEM

Place one foot forward and the opposite foot to the back and slightly out to the side. Count to 10. Increase time up to 60 seconds as tolerated maintaining your balance in this position.

SPLIT STANCE

FOLLOW STEPS 2-8 AS SEEN WITH NARROW BOS AS OUTLINED IN BALANCE PROGRESSION

1. HOLD STEADY OBJECT PROGRESSING TO NO SUPPORT
2. STAND FOR 10-60 SECONDS
3. ARM MOVEMENT
4. TRUNK ROTATION
5. EYES SHUT
6. HEAD TURNS
7. READING
8. **UNSTABLE**

REPEAT ABOVE ON UNSTABLE SURFACE SUCH AS BALANCE PAD, PILLOW, BALANCE DISC, HALF FOARM ROLL OR BOSU.

	_____ Reps _____ Sets _____X Day _____Hold		_____ Reps _____ Sets _____X Day _____Hold
11	Notes:	12	Notes:

TANDEM- SHARPENED ROMBERG STANCE

Place the heel of one foot so that it touches the toes of the other foot. Count to 10. Increase time up to 60 seconds as tolerated maintaining your balance in this position.

TANDEM STANCE

FOLLOW STEPS 2-8 AS SEEN WITH NARROW BOS AS OUTLINED IN BALANCE PROGRESSION

1. HOLD STEADY OBJECT PROGRESSING TO NO SUPPORT
2. STAND FOR 10-60 SECONDS
3. ARM MOVEMENT
4. TRUNK ROTATION
5. EYES SHUT
6. HEAD TURNS
7. READING
8. **UNSTABLE**

REPEAT ABOVE ON UNSTABLE SURFACE SUCH AS BALANCE PAD, PILLOW, BALANCE DISC, HALF FOARM ROLL OR BOSU.

	_____ Reps _____ Sets _____X Day _____Hold		_____ Reps _____ Sets _____X Day _____Hold
13	Notes:	14	Notes:

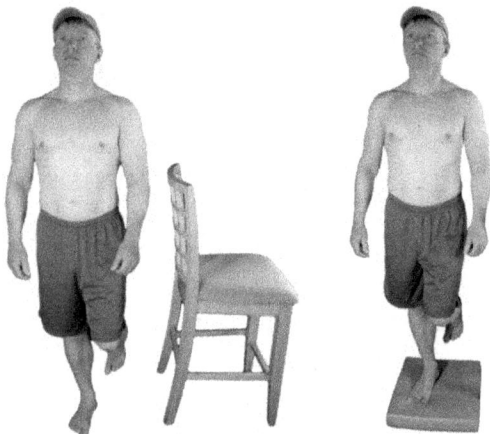

SINGLE LEG STANCE (SLS)

Stand on one foot. Count to 10 > 60 seconds as tolerated maintaining your balance in this position. Maintain a slightly bent knee on the stance side.

SINGLE LEG STANCE

FOLLOW STEPS 2-8 AS SEEN WITH NARROW BOS AS OUTLINED IN BALANCE PROGRESSION

1. HOLD STEADY OBJECT PROGRESSING TO NO SUPPORT
2. STAND FOR 10-60 SECONDS
3. ARM MOVEMENT
4. TRUNK ROTATION
5. EYES SHUT
6. HEAD TURNS
7. READING
8. **UNSTABLE**

REPEAT ABOVE ON UNSTABLE SURFACE SUCH AS BALANCE PAD, PILLOW, BALANCE DISC, HALF FOARM ROLL OR BOSU.

Single Leg Stance (SLS) with Arm and/or Leg Movements- *Progress to Balance Pad*

	_____ Reps _____ Sets _____X Day _____Hold		_____ Reps _____ Sets _____X Day _____Hold
15	Notes:	16	Notes:

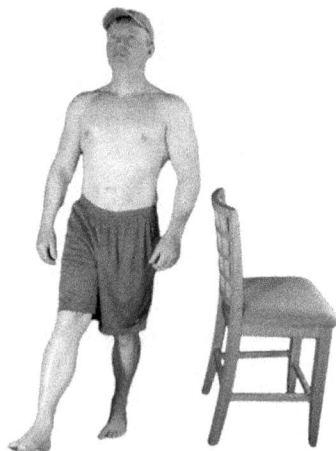

SLS – LEG FORWARD

Stand on one leg and maintain your balance. Hold your leg out in front of your body and then return to the original position. Repeat on opposite side. Maintain a slightly bent knee on the stance side.

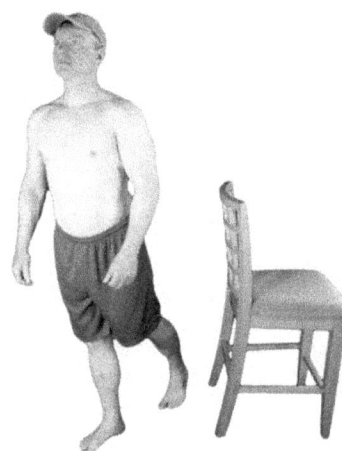

SLS – LEG BACKWARDS

Stand on one leg and maintain your balance. Hold your leg in the back of your body and then return to original position. Repeat on opposite side. Maintain a slightly bent knee on the stance side.

	_____ Reps _____ Sets _____X Day _____Hold		_____ Reps _____ Sets _____X Day _____Hold
17	**Notes:**	**18**	**Notes:**

SLS – LEG FORWARD / OPPOSITE ARM UP

Stand on one leg and maintain your balance. Hold your leg out in front of your body and opposite arm up over your head. Return to the original position. Repeat on opposite side. Maintain a slightly bent knee on the stance side.

SLS – LEG BACKWARDS / OPPOSITE ARM UP

Stand on one leg and maintain your balance. Hold your leg out in front of your body and opposite arm up over your head. Return to the original position. Repeat on opposite side. Maintain a slightly bent knee on the stance side.

	_____ Reps _____ Sets _____X Day _____Hold		_____ Reps _____ Sets _____X Day _____Hold
19	**Notes:**	**20**	**Notes:**

SLS - REACH FORWARD

Stand on one leg and maintain your balance. Reach forward with your opposite arm as far as you can without losing your balance and then return to original position. Repeat on opposite side. Maintain a slightly bent knee on the stance side.

SLS - REACH TWIST

Stand on one leg and maintain your balance. Reach forward and across your body with your opposite arm as far as you can without losing your balance and then return to original position. Repeat on opposite side. Maintain a slightly bent knee on the stance side.

	_____ Reps _____ Sets _____X Day _____Hold
21	Notes:

SINGLE LEG TOE TAP

Start by standing on one leg and maintain your balance. Tap the opposite foot on a slightly raised object, such as a box or balance pad. To progress, increase the height of object, such as a stair step or cone. Can alternate feet or repeat on same side for several repetitions and then repeat on opposite side.

	_____ Reps _____ Sets _____X Day _____Hold
22	Notes:

SINGLE LEG STANCE - CLOCKS

Start by standing on one leg and maintain your balance. Image a clock on the floor where your stance leg is in the center. Lightly touch position 1 as illustrated with the opposite foot. Then return that leg to the starting position. Next, touch position 2 and return. Maintain a slightly bent knee on the stance side.

	_____ Reps _____ Sets _____X Day _____Hold
23	Notes:

BALL ROLLS - HEEL TOE

In a standing position, place one foot on a ball and roll it forward and back in a controlled motion from heel to toe while maintaining your balance.

	_____ Reps _____ Sets _____X Day _____Hold
24	Notes:

BALL ROLLS - LATERAL

In a standing position, place one foot on a ball and roll it side to side in a controlled motion from the inner side of your foot to the outer side of your foot while maintaining your balance.

Squats

	_____ Reps _____ Sets _____ X Day _____ Hold		_____ Reps _____ Sets _____ X Day _____ Hold
25	Notes:	26	Notes:

SQUAT – Can use chair or counter for support and chair behind if needed.

Stand with feet shoulder width apart (in front of a stable support for balance if needed.) Bend your knees and lower your body towards the floor. Your body weight should mostly be directed through the heels of your feet. Return to a standing position. Knees should bend in line with toes and not pass the front of the foot.

SIT TO STAND - Can use armchair to push off if needed

Start by scooting close to the front of the chair. Lean forward at your trunk and reach forward with your arms and rise to standing. (You may use a chair with arms to push off if needed and progress as tolerated).

Use your arms as a counterbalance by reaching forward when in sitting and lower them as you approach standing.

	_____ Reps _____ Sets _____ X Day _____ Hold		_____ Reps _____ Sets _____ X Day _____ Hold
27	Notes:	28	Notes:

SQUATS – WALL WITH BALL

Place either a small ball or therapy ball between you and the wall. Bend your knees and lower your body towards the floor. Return to a standing position. Knees should bend in line with toes and not pass the front of the foot.

SQUATS WITH WEIGHTS

Hold dumbbells or other weights in both hands by your side. Bend your knees and lower your body towards the floor. Return to a standing position. Knees should bend in line with toes and not pass the front of the foot

	_____ Reps _____ Sets _____ X Day _____ Hold		_____ Reps _____ Sets _____ X Day _____ Hold
29	Notes:	**30**	Notes:

MINI SQUAT - UNSTABLE SUPPORT - FOAM PAD

Start with your feet shoulder-width apart, toes pointed straight ahead and standing on a balance pad. Next, bend your knees to approximately 30 degrees of flexion to perform a mini squat as shown. Then, return to original position. Knees should not pass the front of the foot.

SQUATS - SINGLE LEG

While standing on one leg in front of a stable support for assisted balance, bend your knee and lower your body towards the floor. Return to a standing position.
Knees should not pass the front of the foot.

Weight Shifts, Wall Falls, Balance Recovery (Balance Drills)

	_____ Reps _____ Sets _____ X Day _____ Hold		_____ Reps _____ Sets _____ X Day _____ Hold
31	Notes:	**32**	Notes:

SIDE TO SIDE WEIGHT SHIFT
Stand next to stable surface if needed for support.

Keep feet shoulder width apart. Lean from side to side maintaining balance. _May stand in hallway with walls on both sides._
*Advance to using balance pad

FORWARD AND BACKWARDS WEIGHT SHIFTS
Stand next to stable surface if needed for support.

Keep feet shoulder width apart. Lean from body forward and then backwards maintaining balance. _May stand in hallway with wall in front and in back._
*Advance to using balance pad

	_____ Reps _____ Sets _____X Day _____Hold		_____ Reps _____ Sets _____X Day _____Hold
33	Notes:	34	Notes:

SPLIT STANCE WEIGHT SHIFT SIDE TO SIDE
Stand next to stable surface if needed for support.

Stand in a split stance position. Lean side to side maintaining balance. *May stand in hallway with wall on both sides.*

SPLIT STANCE WEIGHT SHIFT FORWARD AND BACKWARDS Stand next to stable surface if needed for support.

Stand in a split stance position. Lean forward and backwards maintaining balance. *May stand in hallway with wall in front and in back.*

	_____ Reps _____ Sets _____X Day _____Hold		_____ Reps _____ Sets _____X Day _____Hold
35	Notes:	36	Notes:

WALL FALLS - FORWARD - BALANCE DRILL

Stand facing wall, a couple feet away from the wall. Slowly and controlled, lean forward towards the wall. Try to control your balance to prevent falling forward. Keep leaning forward gradually until eventually you do lose your balance and fall. Use your arms to catch yourself. Push yourself back upright.

WALL FALLS - LATERAL - BALANCE DRILL

Stand to the side next to a wall, a couple feet away from the wall. Slowly and controlled, lean to the side towards the wall. Try to control your balance to prevent falling sideways. Keep leaning to the side gradually until eventually you do lose your balance and fall. Use your arm to catch yourself. Push yourself back upright.

_____ Reps _____ Sets _____ X Day _____ Hold

37 Notes:

WALL FALLS - BACKWARDS - BALANCE DRILL

Stand facing away from a wall. Slowly and controlled, lean backward towards the wall. Try to control your balance to prevent falling backwards. Keep leaning backwards gradually until eventually you do lose your balance and fall. Use your upper back to catch the fall. Push yourself back upright.

_____ Reps _____ Sets _____ X Day _____ Hold

38 Notes:

WALL FALLS - SINGLE LEG - FORWARD - BALANCE DRILL

Stand on one leg facing a wall, a couple feet away from the wall. Slowly and controlled, lean forward towards the wall. Try to control your balance to prevent falling forward. Keep leaning forward gradually until eventually you do lose your balance and fall. Use your arms to catch yourself. Push yourself back upright.

_____ Reps _____ Sets _____ X Day _____ Hold

39 Notes:

WALL FALLS - SINGLE LEG - LATERAL - BALANCE DRILL

Stand on one leg with a wall a couple feet off to the side of that leg. Slowly and controlled, lean to the side towards the wall. Try to control your balance to prevent falling to the side. Keep leaning gradually towards the wall until eventually you lose your balance and fall. Use your arms to catch yourself. Push yourself back upright.

_____ Reps _____ Sets _____ X Day _____ Hold

40 Notes:

WALL FALLS - SINGLE LEG - MEDIAL - BALANCE DRILL

Stand on one leg with a wall a couple feet off to the opposite side of that leg as shown. Slowly and controlled, lean sideways towards the wall. Try to control your balance to prevent falling to the side. Keep leaning gradually towards the wall until eventually you lose your balance and fall. Use your arms to catch yourself. Push yourself back upright.

_____ Reps _____ Sets _____ X Day _____ Hold

41 Notes:

WALL FALLS - SINGLE LEG - BACKWARDS - BALANCE DRILL

Stand on one leg facing away from a wall. Slowly and controlled, lean backward towards the wall. Try and control your balance to prevent falling backwards. Keep leaning backwards gradually until eventually you do lose your balance and fall. Use your upper back to catch the fall. Push yourself back upright.

_____ Reps _____ Sets _____ X Day _____ Hold

42 Notes:

FALL LATERAL - STEP RECOVERY
Stand next to stable surface if needed for support.

Start in a standing position with feet apart. Slowly lean to the side and try and prevent losing your balance. Continue to lean to the side until eventually you lose your balance and need to take a step to prevent falling.

_____ Reps _____ Sets _____ X Day _____ Hold

43 Notes:

FALL FORWARD - STEP RECOVERY
Stand next to stable surface if needed for support.

Start in a standing position with feet apart. Slowly lean forward and try and prevent losing your balance. Continue to lean forward until eventually you lose your balance and need to take a step to prevent falling.

_____ Reps _____ Sets _____ X Day _____ Hold

44 Notes:

FALL BACKWARD - STEP RECOVERY
Stand next to stable surface if needed for support.

Start in a standing position with feet apart. Slowly lean back and try and prevent losing your balance. Continue to lean backwards until eventually you lose your balance and need to take a step to prevent falling.

LEG EXERCISES > BALANCE > RESISTANCE

SOLID GROUND:
1. **Support:** Hold onto chair, counter, sink or another stationary object
2. **No Support:** Stand next to stable surface if needed for support
3. **Resistance:** Add ankle weights on use elastic band for resistance

UNSTABLE SURFACE: Balance pad, Bosu, Half foam roll, Pillow or Other unstable surface
1. **Support:** Hold onto chair, counter or another stationary object.
2. **No Support:** Stand next to stable surface if needed for support.
3. **Resistance:** Add ankle weights on use elastic band for resistance

Peripheral Neuropathy – See beginning of section for Caution on Unstable Surface

	_____ Reps _____ Sets _____ X Day _____ Hold		_____ Reps _____ Sets _____ X Day _____ Hold
45	Notes:	46	Notes:

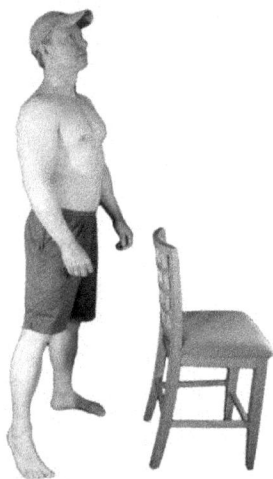

TOE TAP ABDUCTION

Standing upright and move your leg out to the side and tap your toe on the ground. Return to starting position and repeat.

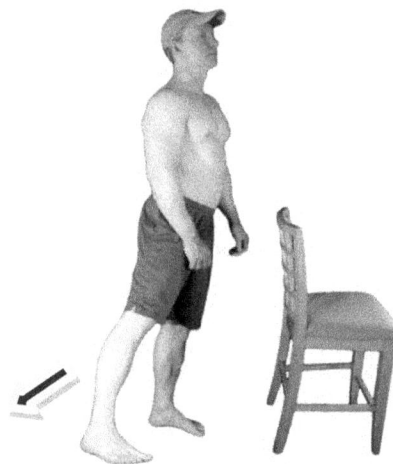

HIP ABDUCTION - STANDING – Can add ankle weights or elastic band.

Standing upright, raise your leg out to the side. Keep your knee straight and maintain your toes pointed forward the entire time. Return to starting position and repeat. Maintain a slow, controlled movement throughout.

_____ Reps _____ Sets _____ X Day _____ Hold		_____ Reps _____ Sets _____ X Day _____ Hold
47	Notes:	**48**	Notes:

HIP EXTENSION – STANDING - Can add ankle weights or band.

Standing upright, balance on one leg and move your other leg in a backward direction. Do not swing the leg and tighten the buttock at end range. Keep your trunk stable and without arching or bending forward during the movement. Return to starting position and repeat. Maintain a slow, controlled movement throughout.

HIP FLEXION - STANDING – STRAIGHT LEG RAISE - Can add ankle weights or band.

Standing upright, balance on one leg and lift your other leg forward with a straight knee as shown. Return to starting position and repeat. Maintain a slow, controlled movement throughout.

_____ Reps _____ Sets _____ X Day _____ Hold		_____ Reps _____ Sets _____ X Day _____ Hold
49	Notes:	**50**	Notes:

HIP / KNEE FLEXION - SINGLE LEG - Can add ankle weights

Standing upright, lift your foot and knee up, set it down. Repeat. Maintain a slow, controlled movement throughout.

STANDING MARCHING- Can add ankle weights

Standing upright, draw up your knee, set it down and then alternate to your other side. Maintain a slow, controlled movement throughout.

	_____ Reps _____ Sets _____ X Day _____ Hold		_____ Reps _____ Sets _____ X Day _____ Hold
51	Notes:	**52**	Notes:

HAMSTRING CURL - Can add ankle weights.

Standing upright, balance on one leg while bending the knee of the opposite leg towards the buttocks. Return to starting position and repeat. Maintain a slow, controlled movement throughout.

TOE RAISES - Can add hand weights.

Standing upright, go up on your toes slowly towards the ceiling and then return to the starting position. Maintain a slow, controlled movement throughout.

	_____ Reps _____ Sets _____ X Day _____ Hold		_____ Reps _____ Sets _____ X Day _____ Hold
53	Notes:	**54**	Notes:

TOE RAISES IR AND ER - Can add hand weights.

IR (Internal Rotation)
Standing upright, rotate feet/legs inward and go up on your toes slowly towards the ceiling and then return to the starting position. Maintain a slow, controlled movement throughout.
ER (External Rotation)
Standing upright, rotate feet/legs outward and go up on your toes slowly towards the ceiling and then return to the starting position.

ONE LEGGED TOE RAISE - Can add hand weights.

Standing upright and balance on one leg. Go up on your toes on the opposite leg towards the ceiling and then return to the starting position. Maintain a slow, controlled movement throughout.

BOSU – Can use chair for stability

_____ Reps _____ Sets _____X Day _____Hold	_____ Reps _____ Sets _____X Day _____Hold
55 Notes:	**56** Notes:

SINGLE LEG BALANCE FORWARD

Stand on a Bosu with one leg and maintain your balance. Hold your opposite leg out in front of your body and then return to original position. Maintain a slightly bent knee on the stance side.

SINGLE LEG BALANCE LATERAL

Stand on a Bosu with one leg and maintain your balance. Hold your opposite leg out to the side of your body and then return to original position. Maintain a slightly bent knee on the stance side.

_____ Reps _____ Sets _____X Day _____Hold	_____ Reps _____ Sets _____X Day _____Hold
57 Notes:	**58** Notes:

SINGLE LEG BALANCE RETRO

Stand on a Bosu Ball with one leg and maintain your balance. Hold your opposite leg back behind your body and then return to original position. Maintain a slightly bent knee on the stance side.

SINGLE LEG STANCE RETROLATERAL

Stand on a Bosu Ball with one leg and maintain your balance. Hold your opposite leg back behind and across your body and then return to original position. Maintain a slightly bent knee on the stance side.

_____ Reps _____ Sets _____X Day _____Hold	_____ Reps _____ Sets _____X Day _____Hold
59 Notes:	**60** Notes:

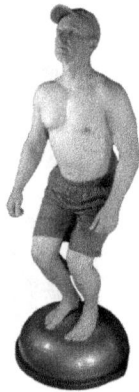

SQUAT

While standing and maintaining your balance on a Bosu, squat and return to a standing position. Knees should bend in line with the 2nd toe and not pass the front of the foot.

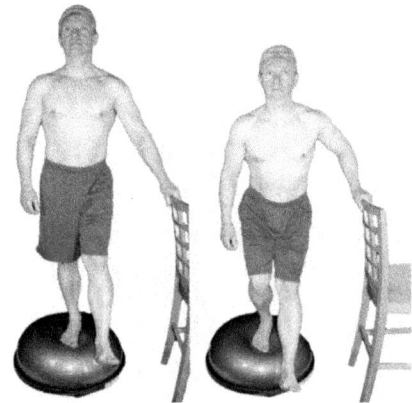

SINGLE LEG SQUAT

While standing and balancing on a Bosu with one leg, bend your knee and lower your body towards the ground. Return to a standing position. Your stance knee should bend in line with the 2nd toe and not pass the front of the foot.

Lunges

_____ Reps _____ Sets _____X Day _____Hold	_____ Reps _____ Sets _____X Day _____Hold
61 Notes:	**62** Notes:

Starting Position

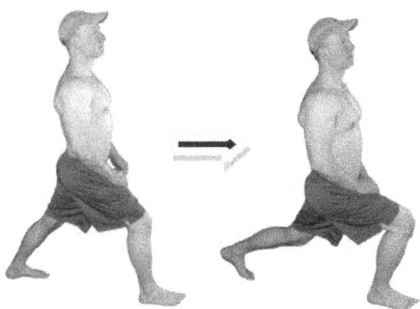

LUNGE – STATIC

Start in standing position with back leg straight and front leg with flexed/bent knee. Lean forward on front knee keeping knee in line with foot and back leg remaining straight. Return to starting position and repeat for several repetitions and then repeat on opposite side. *Make sure front knee does not go past the foot.

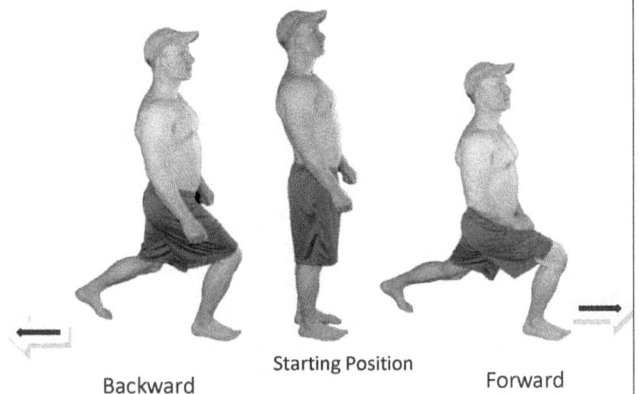

Backward   Starting Position   Forward

LUNGE FORWARD/BACKWARD

Start in standing (*middle picture*).
Backward: Keep one foot planted and step back with the opposite foot. Return to original position - repeat. *Forward:* Keep one foot planted and step forward with the opposite foot. Return to original position - repeat.

DYNAMIC MOVEMENTS

_____ Reps _____ Sets _____X Day _____Hold		_____ Reps _____ Sets _____X Day _____Hold
63	**Notes:**	**64**
	Notes:	

FOUR CORNER MARCHING IN PLACE

Marching in place, move your body clockwise stopping at each corner for several seconds and move to the next corner. After completing the square, march counterclockwise.

FOUR CORNER MARCHING IN PLACE WITH HEAD TURNS

With Head and Body Moving Simultaneously
March in place to four corners, as previous exercise (#63). Move your head and body moving simultaneously as you complete the square.
With Head Turn And Then Body Turn.
March in place to four corners, as previous exercise (#63). Turn head and then body as you complete the square.

_____ Reps _____ Sets _____X Day _____Hold		_____ Reps _____ Sets _____X Day _____Hold
65	**Notes:**	**66**
	Notes:	

WALKING ON HEELS FORWARD AND BACKWARDS – May walk along kitchen counter or wall until feeling steady.

Standing up tall, walk forward on heels. After feeling secure with a forward motion, try walking backwards on heels.

WALKING ON TOES FORWARD AND BACKWARDS – May walk along kitchen counter or wall until feeling steady.

Standing up tall, walk forward on up on toes. After feeling secure with a forward motion, try walking backwards up on toes.

_____ Reps _____ Sets _____ X Day _____ Hold	_____ Reps _____ Sets _____ X Day _____ Hold

67 Notes:

68 Notes:

TANDEM STANCE AND WALK – FORWARD AND BACKWARDS

Maintaining your balance, stand with one foot directly in front of the other so that the toes of one foot touches the heel of the other. Progress by taking steps with your heel touching your toes with each step.
**Progress by walking backwards with your toe touching your heel with each step. Can also add head turns.

RUNNING MAN

Stand and balance on one leg. Lean forward as you bring your other leg back behind you to tap the floor. Bring the same side arm forward as shown during the movement. Return to starting position and repeat.

_____ Reps _____ Sets _____ X Day _____ Hold	_____ Reps _____ Sets _____ X Day _____ Hold

69 Notes:

70 Notes:

HOP STICK - FORWARD

Stand on one leg and then hop forward onto the other leg. Maintain your balance the entire time. Increase the difficulty by hoping forward further or higher.

HOP STICK - BACKWARDS

Stand on one leg and then hop backward onto the other leg. Maintain your balance the entire time. Increase the difficulty by hoping back further or higher.

_____ Reps _____ Sets _____X Day _____Hold	_____ Reps _____ Sets _____X Day _____Hold

71 | Notes:

72 | Notes:

MINI LATERAL LUNGE

Step to the side and balance on the leg. Next return to the original position. Repeat in the opposite direction. Your knees should be bent about 30 degrees.

SIDE STEPPING – May step along kitchen counter or in hallway for support.

Step to the side continuing for length of room or counter – repeat in opposite direction.

_____ Reps _____ Sets _____X Day _____Hold	_____ Reps _____ Sets _____X Day _____Hold

73 | Notes:

74 | Notes:

HOP STICK - LATERAL

Stand on one leg and then hop to the side onto the other leg. Maintain your balance the entire time. Increase the difficulty by hoping to the side further and higher.

SINGLE LEG DEAD LIFT

While standing on one leg, bend forward with arms in front towards the ground as you extend your leg behind you and then return to the original position. Keep your legs straight and maintain your balance the entire time.

_____ Reps _____ Sets _____ X Day _____ Hold	_____ Reps _____ Sets _____ X Day _____ Hold

75 Notes:

76 Notes:

CONE TAPS - SINGLE LEG STANCE

Place 3-5 cones or cups around you as shown. Balance on a slightly bent knee. Lower yourself down to tap the top of a cone with your finger. Return to original position and repeat touching a different cone. Advance exercise with smaller cones/cups and or faster speed.

CONE TAPS - SINGLE LEG STANCE - UNSTABLE

Place 3-5 cones or cups around you. Balance on an unstable surface such as a foam pad with a slightly bent knee. Lower yourself down to tap the top of a cone. Return to original position and repeat touching a different cone. Advance exercise with smaller cones/cups and or faster speed.

_____ Reps _____ Sets _____ X Day _____ Hold	_____ Reps _____ Sets _____ X Day _____ Hold

77 Notes:

78 Notes:

FIGURE 8 AROUND CONES

Set up 4-8 cones on the floor about 12 inches apart, although can vary to increase or decrease difficulty. Weave in and out of cones and then turn and repeat.

FIGURE 8 AROUND CONES – FOOT OR HAND TAP

Follow #75 figure around 4- 8 cones. To increase difficulty, you can tap each cone with your foot or lean over and tap with your hand.

HALF ROLLER (static and dynamic) – FLAT SIDE UP OR DOWN

	_____ Reps _____ Sets _____X Day _____Hold		_____ Reps _____ Sets _____X Day _____Hold
79	Notes:	80	Notes:

BALANCE DOUBLE LEG STANCE - WIDE

Place a half foam roll on the ground in a side-to-side direction. Stand on the foam roll with your feet spread apart and maintain your balance.

BALANCE DOUBLE LEG STANCE - NARROW

Place a half foam roll on the ground in a side-to-side direction. Stand on the foam roll with your feet together and maintain your balance.

	_____ Reps _____ Sets _____X Day _____Hold		_____ Reps _____ Sets _____X Day _____Hold
81	Notes:	82	Notes:

TANDEM STANCE

Place a half foam roll on the ground in a forward-back direction. Stand on the foam roll in tandem stance (with your heel and toe touching as shown) and maintain your balance.

TANDEM WALK

Place a half foam roll on the ground in a forward-back direction. Stand on the foam roll and begin tandem walking (heel-toe pattern walking as shown). Once you get to the end of the roll, either turn around or tandem walk backward.

_____ Reps _____ Sets _____ X Day _____ Hold	_____ Reps _____ Sets _____ X Day _____ Hold

83 Notes:

84 Notes:

SINGLE LEG STANCE - ABDUCTION

Place a half foam roll on the ground in a side-to-side direction. Balance on one leg and move the opposite leg to the side.

SINGLE LEG STANCE - ABDUCTION

Place a half foam roll on the ground in a forward-back direction. Balance on one leg with the opposite leg to the side.

_____ Reps _____ Sets _____ X Day _____ Hold	_____ Reps _____ Sets _____ X Day _____ Hold

85 Notes:

86 Notes:

SINGLE LEG STANCE – FORWARD KICK

Place a half foam roll on the ground in a forward-back direction. Balance on one leg and move the opposite leg forward.

SINGLE LEG STANCE – HAMSTRING CURL

Place a half foam roll on the ground in a forward-back direction. Balance on one leg and with the opposite leg, bend the knee backwards as shown.

	_____ Reps _____ Sets _____ X Day _____ Hold		_____ Reps _____ Sets _____ X Day _____ Hold
87	Notes:	**88**	Notes:

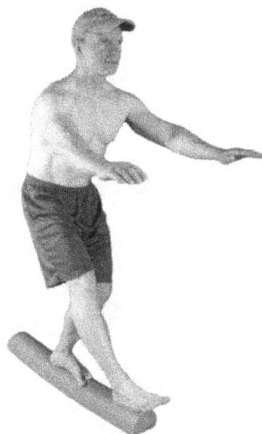

SINGLE LEG SQUAT – LEG FORWARD

Place a half foam roll on the ground in a forward-back direction. Balance on one leg with a slight bend in the supporting knee and move the opposite leg forward. Straighten supporting knee and repeat.

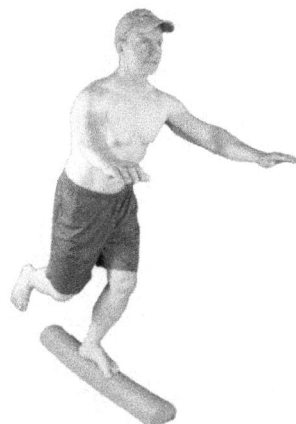

SINGLE LEG SQUAT – LEG BACKWARDS

Place a half foam roll on the ground in a forward-back direction. Balance on one leg with a slight bend in the supporting knee and with the opposite leg, move the leg backwards as shown with bent knee. Straighten supporting knee and repeat.

STAIR STEP – _To progress, increase step height_

	_____ Reps _____ Sets _____ X Day _____ Hold		_____ Reps _____ Sets _____ X Day _____ Hold
89	Notes:	**90**	Notes:

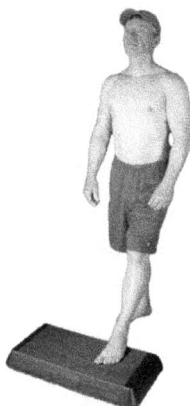

TOE TAP OR HEEL PLACEMENT

While standing with both feet on the floor, place one foot on the top of the step. Next, return the foot back to the floor and then repeat with the other leg.
You can either put your foot up for several repetitions or alternate.

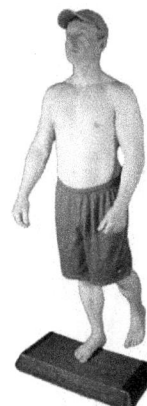

PULL UP FOOT TOUCHES ON STEP

Whie standing with both feet on the ground, put one foot on the step. Push through the foot straightening the knee until the opposite foot is off the ground. Lower the foot back to the starting position. Repeat with the opposite foot for several repetitions.

	_____ Reps _____ Sets _____ X Day _____ Hold
91	**Notes:**

ALTERNATING SUSTAINED FOOT TOUCHES ON STEP

Whie standing with both feet on the ground, put one foot on the step. Push through the foot straightening the knee until the opposite foot is also on the step. Step off backwards to the starting position. Repeat with the opposite foot for several repetitions.

	_____ Reps _____ Sets _____ X Day _____ Hold
92	**Notes:**

STEP UP AND OVER

Step up onto the step and then onto the ground on the other side. Turn around and repeat.
Repeat several repetitions on one side and then the other or alternate legs.

	_____ Reps _____ Sets _____ X Day _____ Hold
93	**Notes:**

FORWARD SWING THROUGH STEP

Step up onto the step without stopping on the top, swing opposite leg through and onto the floor on the other side.

	_____ Reps _____ Sets _____ X Day _____ Hold
94	**Notes:**

SIDE STEPPING

******REPEAT STEPS 89-93 from a side approach******

Agility

EXERCISE Agility/Reactivity/Speed	EXERCISE NUMBER	NOTES
Four Square Drills	1	
Dots	2	
Ladder Drills	3	
Box Drills	4	
Cones	5	
Hurdles	6	

Agility/Reactivity/Speed

According to the Twist Conditioning workbook, "Agility is the ability to link several fundamental movement skills into a multidirectional pattern. Reaction skills are the 'whole body' responsiveness to external stimuli, as well as muscle and joint internal reactivity. Quickness is the ability to explosively initiate movement from a stationary position, as well as shifting the gears of speed". (*Twist, Peter, Twist Agility, Quickness and & Reactivity Workbook, 2009, pg 16*)

Agility is a combination of acceleration, deceleration, coordination, power, strength and dynamic balance. With agility training, always keep your head in a neutral position looking straight ahead no matter which way you turn. "Powerful arm movement during transitional and directional changes is essential in order to reacquire a high rate of speed". (*Brown & Ferrigno, 2005, pp 73-74*)

Agility exercises can be done with cones, hurdles, dots or squares on the floor, box drills, Bosu or ladders. Agility can also be high impact or explosive movements. If you are not comfortable with this in the beginning or have any contraindications, stick with low impact movements. In other words, if you are jumping over hurdles, keep them low to the ground and jump over with one leg leading for low impact and jump with both legs for high impact.

If you are doing box drills or Bosu, please do NOT JUMP off backwards.

AGILITY / SPEED / REACTIVITY

4 Square Drills

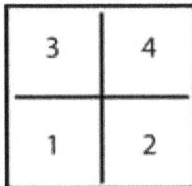
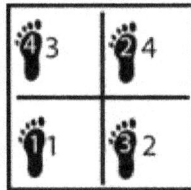
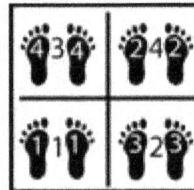
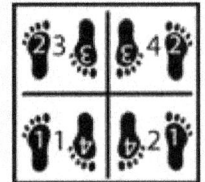

Dots

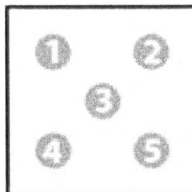
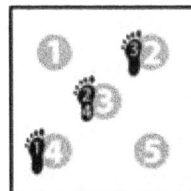
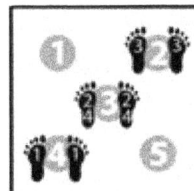
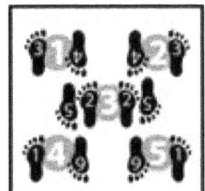

Ladder

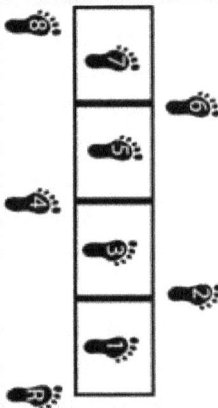
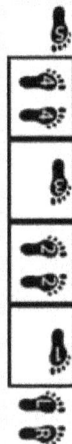
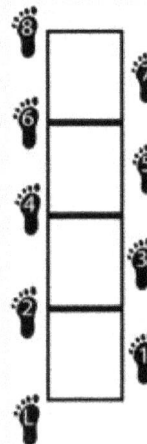
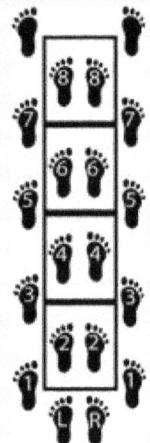

Box Drills – Box should be no higher than the middle of your shin. This can be done on Bosu for balance.

Alt Tap Box With Foot	Down Up Both Feet Together	Quickly Move Side to Side	Down Up Both Feet Together
Switch			

Cones

Hurdles – can run or jump over hurdles

Endurance / Aerobic Capacity

Aerobic - with oxygen: Muscular and Cardiovascular

Many repetitions with sub-maximal weight (weight that is less than the maximum you can lift).

Muscular endurance is the ability of the muscle or group of muscles to sustain repeated contractions against resistance for an extended period of time. This is needed to build muscle. (See *Strengthening*). Cardiovascular endurance is the ability of the heart, lungs and blood vessels to deliver oxygen to working muscles and tissues, as well as the ability of those muscles and tissues to utilize that oxygen. This is needed to help endure long runs or sustained activity, as with biking or running. In short, endurance or aerobic exercises increase the heart rate and respiratory rate.

As far as long-term performance goes, there are two types of muscle fibers that can determine the likelihood of success: slow and fast twitch, which may determine whether you are more likely to be a power-lifter or sprinter (*fast twitch*), or a marathon runner (*slow twitch*). Your ability depends on the distribution of these fibers in the body. In other words, you could have a certain percentage of slow twitch in your biceps, but a different percentage in your quadriceps. There is some controversy over whether you can change the percentage or distribution of these fibers with endurance training or training for a specific event, although you may be able to change the glycolytic capacity.

Type of Fibers	*Slow twitch fibers:* Have a high aerobic capacity and are resistant to fatigue. People that have a higher percentage of slow twitch fibers tend to have better endurance abilities. *Fast twitch fibers:* Contract faster than slow twitch, and thus fatigue faster. People that have a higher percentage of fast twitch fibers tend to have better sprinting or muscle building abilities.

The following research is from the: **MAYO CLINIC**

Mayo Clinic - *https://www.mayoclinic.org/healthy-lifestyle/fitness/in-depth/aerobic-exercise/art-20045541*

Regular aerobic activity, such as walking, bicycling or swimming, can help you live longer and healthier. Need motivation? See how aerobic exercise affects your heart, lungs and blood flow.

How your body responds to aerobic exercise

During aerobic activity, you repeatedly move large muscles in your arms, legs and hips. You'll notice your body's responses quickly.

You'll breathe faster and more deeply. This maximizes the amount of oxygen in your blood. Your heart will beat faster, which increases blood flow to your muscles and back to your lungs.

Your small blood vessels (capillaries) will widen to deliver more oxygen to your muscles and carry away waste products, such as carbon dioxide and lactic acid.

Your body will even release endorphins, natural painkillers that promote an increased sense of well-being.

What aerobic exercise does for your health.

Regardless of age, weight or athletic ability, aerobic activity is good for you. As your body adapts to regular aerobic exercise, you will get stronger and fitter.

Consider the following 10 ways that aerobic activity can help you feel better and enjoy life to the fullest on the next page.

Aerobic activity can help you:

1. **Keep excess pounds at bay**
   Combined with a healthy diet, aerobic exercise helps you lose weight and keep it off.

2. **Increase your stamina**
   You may feel tired when you first start regular aerobic exercise. But over the long term, you'll enjoy increased stamina and reduced fatigue.

3. **Ward off viral illnesses**
   Aerobic exercise activates your immune system in a good way. This may leave you less susceptible to minor viral illnesses, such as colds and flu.

4. **Reduce your health risks**
   Aerobic exercise reduces the risk of many conditions, including obesity, heart disease, high blood pressure, type 2 diabetes, metabolic syndrome, stroke and certain types of cancer.

   Weight-bearing aerobic exercises, such as walking, help decrease the risk of osteoporosis.

5. **Manage chronic conditions**
   Aerobic exercise may help lower blood pressure and control blood sugar. If you have coronary artery disease, aerobic exercise may help you manage your condition.

6. **Strengthen your heart**
   A stronger heart doesn't need to beat as fast. A stronger heart also pumps blood more efficiently, which improves blood flow to all parts of your body.

7. **Keep your arteries clear**
   Aerobic exercise boosts your high-density lipoprotein (HDL), the "good," cholesterol, and lowers your low-density lipoprotein (LDL), the "bad," cholesterol. This may result in less buildup of plaques in your arteries.

8. **Boost your mood**
   Aerobic exercise may ease the gloominess of depression, reduce the tension associated with anxiety and promote relaxation.

9. **Stay active and independent as you age**
   Aerobic exercise keeps your muscles strong, which can help you maintain mobility as you get older. Studies have found that regular physical activity may help protect memory, reasoning, judgment and thinking skills (cognitive function) in older adults and may improve cognitive function in young adults.

10. **Live longer**
    Studies show that people who participate in regular aerobic exercise live longer than those who don't exercise regularly.

Take the first step

Ready to get more active? Great. Just remember to start with small steps. If you've been inactive for a long time or if you have a chronic health condition, get your doctor's OK before you start. When you're ready to begin exercising, start slowly. You might walk five minutes in the morning and five minutes in the evening.
The next day, add a few minutes to each walking session. Pick up the pace a bit, too. Soon, you could be walking briskly for at least 30 minutes a day and reaping all the benefits of regular aerobic activity.

Other options for aerobic exercise could include cross-country skiing, aerobic dancing, swimming, stair climbing, bicycling, jogging, elliptical training or rowing.

(Mayo Clinic - *https://www.mayoclinic.org/healthy-lifestyle/fitness/in-depth/aerobic-exercise/art-20045541*)

Calories

Calorie: A unit of food energy. The word calorie is ordinarily used instead of the more precise, scientific term kilocalorie. A kilocalorie represents the amount of energy required to raise the temperature of a liter of water 1' centigrade at sea level. Technically, a kilocalorie represents 1,000 true calories of energy. *(MedicineNet.com)*

Calories are a measurement tool, like inches or cups. Calories measure the energy a food or beverage provides from the carbohydrate, fat, protein, and alcohol* it contains. Calories give you the fuel or energy you need to work and play – even to rest and sleep! When choosing what to eat and drink, it's important to get the right mix – enough nutrients without too many calories. Paying attention to calories is an important part of managing your weight. The amount of calories you need are different if you want to gain, lose, or maintain your weight. Tracking what and how much you eat, and drink can help you better understand your calorie intake over time. Each person's body may have different needs for calories and exercise. A healthy lifestyle requires balance in the foods you eat, the beverages you drink, the way you do daily activities, adequate sleep, stress management, and in the amount of activity in your daily routine. *(ChooseMyPlate.gov & CDC)*

Example of Activities and Calories Burned *(ChooseMyPlate.gov)*
A 154-pound man who is 5' 10" will use up (burn) about the number of calories listed doing each activity below. Those who weigh more will use more calories; those who weigh less will use fewer calories. The calorie values listed include both calories used by the activity and the calories used for normal body functioning during the activity time.

EXAMPLE	Approximate calories used (burned) by a 154-pound man	
MODERATE physical activities:	In 1 hour	In 30 minutes
Hiking	370	185
Light gardening/ yard work	330	165
Dancing	330	165
Golf (walking and carrying clubs)	330	165
Bicycling (less than 10 mph)	290	145
Walking (3.5 mph)	280	140
Weight training (general light workout)	220	110
Stretching	180	90
VIGOROUS physical activities:	In 1 hour	In 30 minutes
Running/ jogging (5 mph)	590	295
Bicycling (more than 10 mph)	590	295
Swimming (slow freestyle laps)	510	255
Aerobics	480	240
Walking (4.5 mph)	460	230
Heavy yard work (chopping wood)	440	220
Weightlifting (vigorous effort)	440	220
Basketball (vigorous)	440	220

References

Also, Some Good Books, Websites & DVD'

ACE Idea Fitness Journal*: Martina M. Cartwright, PhD, RD http://www.ideafit.com/fitness-library/protein-today-are-consumers-getting-too-much-of-a-good-thing?ACE_ACCESS=ebec6bcf61abff08f7b1d8b27c555758*

ACE Senior Fitness Manual, *American Council on Exercise* (2014)

American Physical Therapy Association, (APTA), 2007. *Basic Science for Animal Physical Therapy: Canine, 2nd edition*

Arleigh J Reynolds, DVM, PhD - *www.absasleddogracing.org.uk/newgang/src/gangline/role.htm*

Australian Institute of Sports - *http://www.ausport.gov.au*

BodyBuilder.com

Brown & Ferrigno, (2005). *Training for Speed, Agility and Quickness*, Champaign, IL: Human Kinetics.

Bryant, C & Green, D, editors (2003), *Ace Personal Trainer Manual, 3rd ed.*, San Diego, CA: American Council on Exercise (ACE)

ChooseMyPlate.gov

Examine.com

ExRx.net

Feher & Szunyoghy (1996). *Cyclopedia Anatomicae,* Tess Press

Gillette, R (2002). Temperature Regulation of the Dog. Retrieved June 2011 from *http://www.sportsvet.com/11Nwsltr.PDF*

Gillette, R (2008). *Feeding the Canine Athlete for Optimal Performance.* Retrieved September 25, 2008 from *www.sports vet.com/Art3.html.*

Glucose (Wikipedia) - *http://en.wikipedia.org/wiki/Glucose*

Glycemic Index (Wikipedia) - *http://en.wikipedia.org/wiki/Glycemic_index*

LiveStrong.com

Mayo Clinic - *https://www.mayoclinic.org/healthy-lifestyle/fitness/in-depth/aerobic-exercise/art-20045541*

MedicineNet.com

Myofascial Release: (Wikipedia) - https://en.wikipedia.org/wiki/Myofascial_release

Rikli, Roberta and Jones, Jessie (2013) *Senior Fitness Test Manual, 2nd Ed.,*

Strength Training: (Wikipedia) *http://en.wikipedia.org/wiki/Strength_training*

Twist, Peter (2009). *Twist Agility, Quickness and & Reactivity Workbook.* British Columbia: Twist Conditioning, Inc. University of Maryland Medical Center.com

Workout Australia

Thank You to:

My Husband
Model
For his support through my battle with cancer and while writing this and previous books.
Also, for the patience and hours he put in modeling for this book.

My Daughter
For giving me artistic inspiration and providing artwork for my previous books.

My Grandchildren
Just Because

God
For giving me the strength to overcome cancer and the wisdom to write these books.

Certifications, Continuing Education and License

Physical Therapist Assistant – L/PTA – 30 years in both Home Therapy and Short-Term Rehab facilities

ACE Certified Personal Trainer – CPT
- Functional Training Specialist
- Therapeutic Exercise Specialist
- Senior Fitness Specialist
- Nutrition and Fitness Specialist

©Klose Education
- Certified Lymphedema Therapist – CLT
- Strength After Breast Cancer – Strength ABC
- Breast Cancer Rehabilitation

©Cancer Exercise Specialist Institute – CETI
- Cancer Exercise Specialist – CES
- Breast Cancer Recovery BOSU(R) Specialist Advanced Qualification
- Pilates Mat Certificate

©MedFit
- Medical Fitness Specialist
- Parkinson's Disease Fitness Specialist
- Arthritis Fitness Specialist

©Pink Ribbon Program

©The BioMechanics Method - Corrective Exercise Specialist

©ISSA - DNA-Based Fitness Coach